Tai Chi Wu Style

Tai Chi Wu Style

Advanced Techniques for Internalizing Chi Energy

Mantak Chia
and
Andrew Jan

Destiny Books
Rochester, Vermont • Toronto, Canada

Destiny Books
One Park Street
Rochester, Vermont 05767
www.DestinyBooks.com

Destiny Books is a division of Inner Traditions International

Library of Congress Cataloging-in-Publication Data
Chia, Mantak, 1944–
  Tai chi, wu style : advanced techniques for internalizing chi energy / Mantak Chia and Andrew Jan.
    p. cm.
  Includes bibliographical references and index.
  ISBN 978-1-59477-471-3 (pbk.) — ISBN 978-1-62055-005-2 (e-book)
  1. Tai chi. 2. Exercise. I. Jan, Andrew. II. Title.
  RM727.T34C45 2013
  613.7'148—dc23

                                                            2012027660

Printed and bound in the United States by Versa Press, Inc.

10   9   8   7   6   5   4   3   2   1

Text design by Priscilla Baker and layout by Virginia Scott Bowman
This book was typeset in Janson Text with Present, Futura, and Sho used as display typefaces

Photographs by Sopitnapa Promnon
Illustrations by Udon Jandee

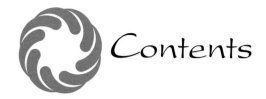

Contents

Acknowledgments

The Universal Tao Publications staff involved in the preparation and production of *Tai Chi Wu Style* extend our gratitude to the many generations of Taoist masters who have passed on their special lineage, in the form of an unbroken oral transmission, over thousands of years. This book is dedicated to the Wu masters of Mantak Chia and Andrew Jan. They are Eddie Yee, John Yuen, Liu Hong-Chi, Kwong Ken-Yue, and Chen Tin-Hung.

We offer our eternal gratitude and love to our parents and teachers for their many gifts to us. Remembering them brings joy and satisfaction to our continued efforts in presenting the Universal Healing Tao system. As always, their contribution has been crucial in presenting the concepts and techniques of the Universal Healing Tao.

We wish to thank the thousands of unknown men and women of the Chinese healing arts who developed many of the methods and ideas presented in this book.

We thank the many contributors essential to this book's final form: the editorial and production staff at Inner Traditions/Destiny Books for their efforts to clarify the text and produce a handsome new edition of the book and Gail Rex for her line edit of the new edition.

We wish to thank the following people for their assistance in producing the earlier editions of this book: Bob Zuraw for sharing his kindness, healing techniques, and Taoist understandings; Colin Drown for his editorial work and writing contributions, as well as his ideas for the cover; Otto Thamboon for his artistic contributions to the revised edition of this book; and our senior instructors, Walter and Jutta Kellenberger, for their insightful contributions to the revised edition. Special thanks to Charles Morris for inspiring and reorganizing the book, without whom the book would not have come to be.

A special thanks goes to our Thai production team: Hirunyathorn Punsan, Saysunee Yongyod, Udon Jandee, and Saniem Chaisam.

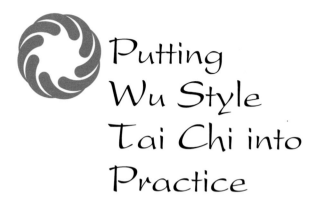

Putting Wu Style Tai Chi into Practice

The practices described in this book have been used successfully for thousands of years by Taoists trained by personal instruction. Readers should not undertake the practice without receiving personal transmission and training from a certified instructor of the Universal Healing Tao, since certain of these practices, if done improperly, may cause injury or result in health problems. This book is intended to supplement individual training by the Universal Healing Tao and to serve as a reference guide for these practices. Anyone who undertakes these practices on the basis of this book alone does so entirely at his or her own risk.

The meditations, practices, and techniques described herein are not intended to be used as an alternative or substitute for professional medical treatment and care. If any readers are suffering from illnesses based on mental or emotional disorders, an appropriate professional health care practitioner or therapist should be consulted. Such problems should be corrected before you start training.

Neither the Universal Healing Tao nor its staff and instructors can be responsible for the consequences of any practice or misuse of the information contained in this book. If the reader undertakes any exercise without strictly following the instructions, notes, and warnings, the responsibility must lie solely with the reader.

This book does not attempt to give any medical diagnosis, treatment, prescription, or remedial recommendation in relation to any human disease, ailment, suffering, or physical condition whatsoever.

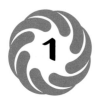

History of the Wu Style

Wu style Tai Chi Chi Kung is one of many styles of Tai Chi that are practiced around the world today. It evolved from the popular Yang style, and indeed it was considered a part of that style until the early twentieth century.

HOW THE WU STYLE
EVOLVED FROM THE YANG STYLE

The founder of the Wu style was a practitioner named Chuan Yu (1834–1902). He learned the art from the Yang master Yang Pan-Hou (1837–1892), the second son of Yang Lu-Chan (1799–1872). The Chuan Yu family were of Manchurian descent rather than Han Chinese, and it is thought that Chuan Yu adopted the Wu name to be better accepted by the dominant Han Chinese population.[1] Wen Zee suggests that the Wu name came from the sound of Chuan Yu's Manchurian name.[2] For the remainder of this text, Chuan Yu will be referred to as Wu Chuan-Yu.*

---

*The Wu name should not be confused with another Tai Chi style that originated with Li Yi-Yu (1832–1892). Because Li Yi-Yu learned from Wu Yu-Hsiang (1812–1880), the Wu name is sometimes used to describe this style, though it is also called the Hao style to avoid confusion. Like Wu Chuan-Yu's master Yang Pan-Hou, Wu Yu-Hsiang also received teachings from Yang Lu-Chan.

Initially, the teachings of Wu Chuan-Yu were not considered separate from the Yang styles. The separation came about in the early twentieth century when a secretary general of the Tai Chi Association, Chu Ming-Yi, was repeatedly thrown in a Push Hands demonstration. In his humiliation he withdrew his support for the Yang style and promoted Wu Chuan-Yu's son instead.[3]

Wu Chuan-Yu was a captain in the imperial guard of the Qing Emperor Guang Xu. At that time, the uniforms of the imperial guard were heavy and elaborate—throwbacks to the form and function of earlier times (fig. 1.1). This garb may have been an external impetus that contributed to a break from the flamboyant Yang style; the heavy imperial robes went all the way down to the knees and hence prevented long stances and fully extended arms.[4] Yang Lu-Chan therefore modified the traditional Yang style to teach Wu Chuan-Yu the Small-Frame Yang style.

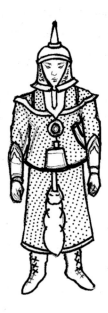

Fig. 1.1. Manchurian warrior garb inhibited wide stances and fully extended arms.

Small-Frame Yang Style

The small-frame styles that exist today are few, including the Yang, Wu, Hao, and Sun styles. There is not a lot of literature about them, but in essence they all exhibit a drift toward more natural stances. This drift reflects a few different principles.

The first principle is that of *fa song*.* While *fa song* is generally translated as "to relax," this is an incomplete translation. A more accurate definition would describe *fa song* as a drift from the outward to the inward—from impressive appearance to alignment with one's internal energies. The mind and senses are turned inward and a new truth of governance is discovered. The practitioner is no longer directed by external impositions but by what unfolds from the inside out.

The second principle is that there is a drift toward finding the best shape and movement form to mimic the natural flow of jin/discharge power. In the classic Yang large-frame stance, the arms are long and the back is straight. This is not conducive to the passage of jin through the spine.

The third principle is that aging is a process of contraction while youth represents growth and extension. With aging, the range of movements of joints and the length of muscles diminish. Therefore, as a master progresses in both proficiency and age, the form tends to become small.

As a consequence of these three principles (*song*, jin, and contracting in aging) the Yang small frame shows a shorter stance, higher postures, less extension and range of the arms, and a slight leaning forward of the postures in attacking forms. The Universal Healing Tao Yang Form typifies these small-frame features. It represents a drift away from the orthodox Yang stance with extended arms to a form that allows the passage of jin and chi from the earth through the legs, spine, and arms. This passage of chi is why this form is referred to as a Tai Chi Chi Kung form rather than just an abbreviated Yang Tai Chi form: it is defined by the passage of chi rather than by a precise outward form.

The Yang style small frame was also displayed by Yang Lu-Chan's other son, Yang Jian (1839–1917). This was passed to Yang Shan-Hou

---

*Fa song is also spelled *fang sung* in the pinyin system of transliteration.

(1860–1932),[5] who cultivated a small frame as well. His style displayed an upright posture and fluid interchanges as well as the small stances.* The small frame was also promulgated by Wu Yu-Hsiang (1812–1890), Li Yi-Yu (1833–1892), Hao style, and Sun Lu-Tang (1861–1932).

Fast Tai Chi

One of the forms of Yang style Tai Chi is Fast Tai Chi. Although this practice is sometimes referred to as Small-Frame Tai Chi, this is a misnomer. Fast Tai Chi and Small-Frame Tai Chi emphasize different aspects of the art.

The Yang Fast Frame (also called the "Discharge Form") can be performed in either a small or large frame. In either case, it emphasizes real-life speed. The slow form developed because it encouraged the foundation principles of Fa Jin, which can only be cultivated with a calm mind and relaxed body. But in Fast Tai Chi, the slow forms have been internalized and can be demonstrated with greater speed. However, Fast Tai Chi forms do not usually replicate the slow forms; they have their own unique routines.

Fast Tai Chi exists in the Wu style. Footage is available of Ma Yueh-Liang (1901–1999)[†] doing a fast form: it appears to be segments of the long form reordered and displayed in real martial time.

THE NORTHERN SCHOOL

The next step in the evolution of the Wu form is the further development from the Small-Frame Yang style to what we generally see in the world today.

We know that Wu Chuan-Yu modified the Yang form to create the Wu form. Some of the innovations he was known for include using

---

*Demonstration of this form can be seen by Yan Shan-Hou's student Zhang Fu-Chen on YouTube; viewed November 2010.
†Ma Yueh-Liang was the husband of Wu Ying-Hua, who was a daughter of Wu Jian-Chuan.

softness to appear as weakness to someone not trained in this style[6] and the focus on "neutralizing" an opponent's force.* Wu Chuan-Yu developed and taught his style—which became known as the Northern Wu school—in Beijing. His lineage there passed through Wang Mao-Zhai (1862–1940), Yang Yu-Ting (1887–1982), Wang Pei-Shang (1919–2004), and Li Bing-Ci (1929–   ).

Wang Mao-Zhai (1862–1940) was the leader of the initial Wu Northern style group in Beijing (fig. 1.2). Footage of later students Wang Pei-Sheng, Yang Yu-Ting, and Li Bing-Ci clearly shows a small frame and the peculiar hand movement called Brush Knee.† (This movement includes beginning the palm strike close to the ear, with the wrist flexed and internally rotated initially. Upon the actual strike, some externally rotate the palm.)

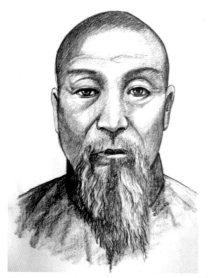

Fig. 1.2. Wang Mao-Zhai

Wang Pei-Sheng performs his routine particularly slowly and demonstrates his thoroughness with each form. He had a reputation for having the best understanding of the applications for each posture,

---

Neutralizing is a term used in Push Hands whereby any attacking force is dissipated. Wu Chuan-Yu had the ability to receive an incoming force, follow it, divert it into the earth, and then convert it to another force.
†Footage of these students and many others can be easily viewed on the internet.

and shared this understanding in an excellent text on the Northern Wu style.* His book provides in-depth descriptions and drawings of each form and its applications.

Yang Yu-Ting has a definite visible power to his form. He was proficient in the three main internal martial arts—Tai Chi, Ba Gua, and Hsying Yi Chuan. He held the post of vice chairman of the Beijing Martial Arts Association. Li Bing-Ci created the official 45-form competition routine for the Chinese Wushu Association, which promoted the Northern style.[7]

THE SOUTHERN SCHOOL
Wu Jian-Chuan

Wu Chuan-Yu's son Wu Jian-Chuan (1870–1942) moved south to Shanghai in 1928 and set up the Wu Southern school (fig. 1.3). Wu Jian-Chuan's reputation quickly spread, and he was appointed to the Board of the Shanghai Martial Arts Association.

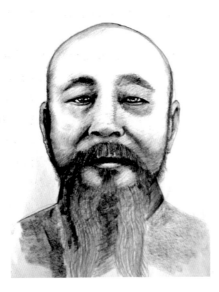

Fig. 1.3. Wu Jian-Chuan

---

*See Wang Pei-Sheng and Zeng Wei-Qi, *Wu Style Taijiquan: A Detailed Course for Health and Self Defence and Teachings of Three Famous Masters in Beijing* (Hong Kong: Hai Feng Publishing Co., 1983).

In the pictures on page 8, which have been redrawn from archival photos, Wu Jian-Chuan performs the single-handed palm strike at the end of the Bird's Tail (fig. 1.4), Single Whip (fig. 1.5), and Flying Oblique (fig. 1.6).

Surprisingly, the frame of Wu Jian-Chuan is larger than expected. This suggests that both a large and a small frame existed at this stage in the evolution of the Wu style. Alternatively, the small frame may have developed in subsequent generations, or it's possible that Wu Jian-Chuan exaggerated the postures for the sake of still photography.

There is actual footage of one of Wu Jian-Chuan's students, Zhu Min-Yi, recorded in 1937 in Shanghai. Analysis of Zhu Min-Yi's form may explain the seemingly large frame displayed by Wu Jian-Chuan. The video footage shows the following characteristics: a small frame, the pace is relatively quick compared to the Northern school, the palms are more Yang in style, and he leads with the heel of his palm. Together, these elements of style support the conclusion that Wu Jian-Chuan exaggerated and enlarged the frame for the sake of the still photographs. The sequence of moves has some variation from the 83-posture sequence of Wu Chuan-Yu's form, which was documented by Yang Yu-Ting in 1947.[8]

Wu Jian-Chuan taught many students. Some of the best known are: Wu Gong-Yi (1900–1970), Zhu Min-Yi, Chen Win-Kwong, Ma Yueh-Liang, and Wu Jian-Chuan's eldest daughter, Wu Ying-Hua (1907–1996). Wu Ying-Hua was the most celebrated of Wu Jian-Chuan's children. She married Ma Yueh-Liang (1901–1998), and the two shared their teachings widely around the globe and in their publications. They passed the art to their son Ma Jiang-Biao (1941–   ).

There is footage available of Wu Ying-Hua.* It reveals less extreme wrist flexion and proximity to the ear in the preparation for the palm strike of the Brush Knee form. It is a fluid, small frame without extreme slanting of the spine—closer to a boxing system and the Sun Lu-Tan and Hao styles.

---

*See Wu Ying-Hua on YouTube; viewed December 2010.

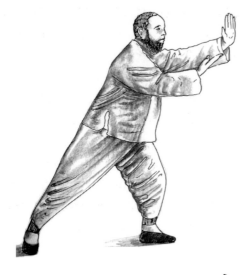

Fig. 1.4. Wu Jian-Chuan performing the single-handed palm strike. Observe the slanted spine and moderate-size frame.

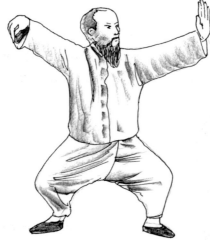

Fig. 1.5. Low stance in the Single Whip

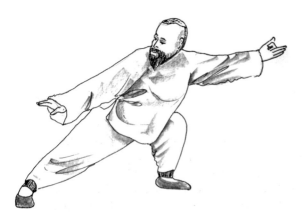

Fig. 1.6. Large frame and long arms in the Flying Oblique

Wu Gong-Yi had a son Wu Ta-Kuei (1923–1972)—a fierce and apparently undefeated fighter—whose eldest son is Eddie Wu Kwong-Yu (1946–   ), the current "gatekeeper" and head of the Wu Southern style. His disciple Eddie Yee taught Mantak Chia the Wu long form, the short form, the sword, the knife, Push Hands, and self-defense techniques. He initiated Mantak Chia into the Wu family circle and taught him the secret inner Tai Chi principles.*

Not that much is written about Chen Win-Kwong, except that he was certainly part of the inner circle of Wu Jian-Chuan's disciples in Hong Kong. He transformed his health through practice and eventually had a reputation as the greatest master in Canton.[9]

Chen Tin-Hung (1930–2005)

Chen Tin-Hung was a nephew of Chen Win-Kwong (fig. 1.7). He was born in Guandong province but lived most of his life in Hong Kong, where he developed a renowned reputation as a full-contact

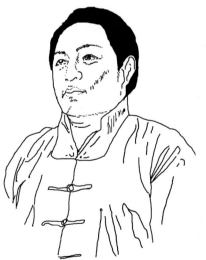

Fig. 1.7. Chen Tin-Hung

---

*Dr. Andrew Jan received teachings predominantly via the Southern lineage that descends through Chen Win-Kwong. He has received direct teachings from Chen Tin-Hung (1930–2005), Ken Yue-Kwong (Rocky) (1934–   ), and John Yuen. These teachings included the long form, Push Hands, boxing, sword, and spear. While living in Beijing he also learned Li Bing-Ci's 45-posture competition form from Liu Hong-Chi.

fighter and won several competitions in the South East Asia region. He wrote several books and also produced a movie, *The Shadow Boxer.*

Chen Tin-Hung fused his boxing skills with internal arts and renamed his style "Wu Tang" Tai Chi. According to Rocky Kwong and other sources, this was done to honor the arts that originated from the Wu Tang Mountain—the legendary home of the immortal Chan San-Feng. However, there is no doubt that Chen Tin-Hung's long Tai Chi form and Push Hands practice belong to the Southern Wu lineage. His book *Wu Tan Tai Chi Chuan* (which includes boxing and martial applications) openly states that "the present book is based on the Wu style."[10] However, the boxing system was most likely developed by Chen Tin-Hung himself and was probably not passed down from Wu Jian-Chuan and Chen Win-Kwong.*

Chen Tin-Hung also introduced a round long form. This form includes silk-reeling types of movements in addition to postures like Seven Stars, Brush Knee, White Crane Spreads Its Wings, Parry and Punch, and so on. This combination of ongoing circular movements (perhaps remnants of the Chen style) with a classic square form gives the whole form a new dimension. Like many of the Southern school videos, it shows a quick pace for the long form.†

Chen Tin-Hung's best-known students abroad include Dan Docherty in the United Kingdom and Rocky Kwong in Australia. Rocky Kwong immigrated to Australia in 1960 after completing ten years of training with Chen Tin-Hung in Hong Kong. He began teaching a handful of students in his restaurant in Boronia, Victoria, around 1969. His reputation rapidly grew, and multiple clubs supervised by Kwong and his key disciples appeared throughout Victoria. Together, they formed the Wu Federation of Australia, which incorporated his disciples and their students. Rocky moved to Western Australia in the 1980s and since then has run multiple classes and taught hundreds of students.

---

*See chapters 7 and 8 in this book for a more detailed discussion of this fused boxing style.
†See YouTube; viewed June 2010.

SUMMARY OF THE WU STYLE

The most notable characteristics of the Wu style—as distinct from the Yang style—are the small frame and the variation in certain postures, as well as in the sequence. These changes are generally common to both Northern school and Southern school practitioners. The only documented exception is in the photographs of Wu Jian-Chuan.

As a general rule, the older the master the smaller the frame. Another general characteristic is that all practitioners exhibit a forward-slanted spine, because this position allows the easier passage of jin through the spine and structure.

Variations occur between the various Northern and Southern sequences; however the similarities in postures and forms are significant enough for them all to be considered part of the same Wu style Tai Chi. The majority of Wu practitioners de-emphasize the heel strike component of the palm strike. In the Wu standard (square) style, the palm begins close to the ear and the wrist is flexed and facing inward. This is more exaggerated in the Northern style, whose practitioners often add a lateral rotation to the palm strike as well. They prefer a slow speed, while the Southern school often performs at quicker rates. Note that this fast speed is different from the Fast Tai Chi forms, which involve a separate sequence.

A brief summary of the Wu forms commonly taught throughout the world include:

Yang Long Form: 108
Long Wu Northern Form: 83
Southern Form (Wu Gong-Tsao): 108
Shanghai Wu Form: 89
Chen Tin-Hung's Long Square Form: 118
Wei Pei-Sheng: 37
Li Bing Ci's Competition Form: 45
Mantak Chia's Short Form: 9

Despite the variation in total number of forms, there are only about 37 individual forms or postures in the Wu style. These include:

1. Preparation
2. Bend Down
3. Grasp the Bird's (Swallow's) Tail
4. Single Whip
5. Flying Oblique
6. Lift Hand and Step Forward (Up)
7. White Crane (Stork) Spreads Its Wings
8. Brush Knee (Twist Step)
9. Play (Stroke) the Lute (Pi Pa or Seven Stars)
10. Advance (Step Up), Parry, and Punch
11. Shutting a Door (Apparent Closing)
12. Embrace Tiger and Return to Mountain
13. Cross Hands
14. Fist under Elbow
15. Step Back and Repulse Monkey
16. Needle at the Sea Bottom
17. Fan through the Back
18. Turn Body and Swing Fist (Strike)
19. Wave Hands in Clouds
20. Pat the Horse High
21. Toe Kick (Kick Out in a Curve)
22. Heel Kick
23. Step Forward and Punch Low (Down or Groin)
24. Turn Body and Swing Fist (Strike)
25. (Step Back) Strike Tiger
26. Boxing (Double Wind) the Ears
27. Parting the Wild Horse's Mane
28. Fair Lady Works the Shuttle
29. Dodge (Crouch) and Kick
30. Snake Creeps Down
31. Golden Cock Stands on One Leg

32. Slap the Face (Palm Strike)
33. Cross (Turn Body) and Single Hand Sweep Lotus Leg
34. Step Back to Ride (Astride) Tiger
35. Draw the Bow to Shoot the Tiger
36. Turn Body and Sweep (Double) Lotus
37. Closing (Completion)

The Universal Healing Tao form is an abbreviated form that includes the first eight moves listed above and a closing form, making a total of nine forms. This short form has the advantage of allowing students to gain the internal benefits without having to first learn a

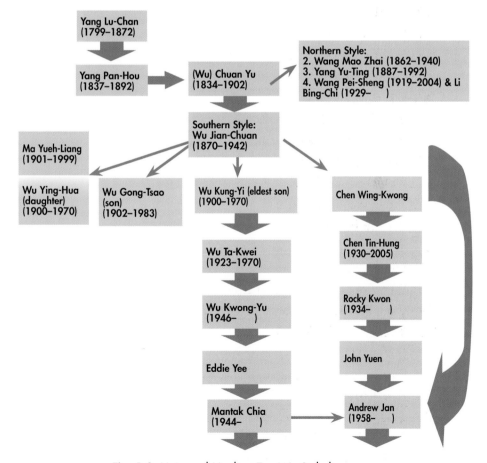

Fig. 1.8. Universal Healing Tao Wu Style lineage

long form. The painstaking process of learning a long from can initially slow down the health and power benefits that come from mastering the movements of chi and jin. After accomplishing the short form, many students choose to advance their studies by embarking on a long form.

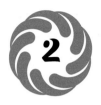

Why Practice Wu Style Tai Chi Chi Kung?

All Taoist arts have a root in alchemy, and all have a positive effect on health, mind, and spirit. Tai Chi in particular is a powerful way to train the body and improve one's physical and spiritual health. This chapter will explore some of the scientific views of Tai Chi as it relates to physical health and will break down the differences among Tai Chi styles.

TAI CHI AND HEALTH

Research conducted around the globe has shown that Tai Chi can improve health. However, many proponents of Tai Chi feel that the research does not reveal the true potential of this practice for healing. It is true that research into areas of Asian medicine such as Tai Chi and acupuncture remains problematic. Firstly, there is not a financial incentive to collaborate and promote these disciplines. Second, most of the good-quality trials are done over 12–16 weeks, which most experts would agree is not enough time. In fact, many

Tai Chi teachers suggest that the benefits of Tai Chi don't really begin to accrue until after a year of practice. Master Wu Tu-Nan (born 1884 and lived more than one hundred years) states, "Generally after learning and practicing in such a manner for a year or so, the movements of these students become much more coordinated and flowing, their health noticeably improves."[1]

Wang Chen-Chen criticizes the design of some studies that have been performed in Asia as nonrandomized controlled trials, retrospective studies, or cohort studies. Others are likely to have publication bias.*[2] Studies performed in the West are supposedly of a higher standard and have included randomized trials. Many of these studies have compared Tai Chi to recognized alternative exercise programs such as hydrotherapy, balance programs, nonintervention, and strength exercises and have been published in highly regarded mainstream journals as well as in alternative ones.

Despite the problems with researching Tai Chi, the evidence from such trials is generally positive. One systematic review of the evidence concluded that "Tai Chi appears to have physiological and psychological benefits and also appears to be safe and effective in promoting balance control, flexibility, and cardiovascular fitness in older persons with chronic conditions."[3] An article in the *Journal of Cardiopulmonary Rehabilitation* found that "recent research has reported improvements in cardio-respiratory function, balance and postural stability, fall prevention and stress reduction."[4] In addition, a *Cochrane Review* on rheumatoid arthritis reported that "there is 'silver' level evidence that Tai Chi improves the range of motion of the ankle, hip, and knee in people with rheumatoid arthritis."[5]

---

*Nonrandomized trials compare Tai Chi to another treatment modality, but selection into the Tai Chi group is not randomized and therefore is likely to be biased. Publication bias occurs when only positive results are published. Many reputable journals now ask that trials be registered prior to beginning of trial to avoid this. Retrospective studies look at those patients who do well and then analyze the data retrospectively. Cohort studies compare one group (for instance, Tai Chi practitioners) and to a similarly aged group of people who don't practice.

Researchers have looked at the health benefits of Tai Chi under the following categories of health and aging.

> **Neurologic:** depression, balance, fall reduction, gait, dizziness reduction, stress reduction, sleep quality, pain levels, and visual-motor integration
>
> **Cardiovascular:** hypertension, microcirculation, postural hypotension
>
> **Respiratory:** peak oxygen uptake and efficiency of volume flow
>
> **Musculoskeletal:** range of movement, ease of movement, muscle strength, bone loss reduction, and posture
>
> **Immune function:** reduction in the occurrence of shingles, improving T-cell function
>
> **Hormonal:** estrogen and testosterone levels
>
> **Overall health:** quality of life

Western medicine is currently mature enough to consider any modality of healing that can produce a positive and measurable outcome, but it is slow to encourage investment or a change of established practice. It doesn't at this stage have a model or paradigm to explain the alleged benefits of Tai Chi and may simply see it as a combination of appropriately graded mechanical exercises linked within a supportive and positive community. For the skeptics, improvements in function may be dismissed as consequences of the placebo effect. One researcher seems to miss the point altogether when she says, "The positive effects of Tai Chi may solely be due to its relaxing and meditative aspects."[6] We hope the reader will understand that these are vital aspects of the practice as well as very important mechanisms of its therapeutic efficacy.

One of the beauties of Tai Chi is that it should "do no harm." This is similar to the foundational principle stipulated by Hippocrates in the fifth century BCE. Tai Chi as a therapy can be contrasted with hazardous invasive procedures and potentially toxic medicines. With Tai Chi, patients can take control of their condition and continue generating positive effects after training sessions. These can take the form of lifestyle changes, dietary changes, stretching, meditation, and so on. The initial benefits are accessed through the support of the teacher but thereafter are best carried on by the patient.

The Taoist or traditional Chinese medicine approach offers some explanations as to how Tai Chi improves health. Its benefits derive, in part, from its effect on posture, the involvement of spirit, emotional health, its integration with community, opportunity for improvement over centuries, and connection with Taoism as a philosophy and religion.

Tai Chi moves the student or patient toward an ideal posture. Bad posture is a reflection of accumulated tension in various parts of the body. One common site of this tension includes the cervical and upper thoracic spine, which results in the head protruding forward and a hump developing at the base of the neck. In tandem with this the shoulders are held high and tightness develops in the shoulder girdle, giving rise to impingement syndromes like painful arc and frozen shoulders.

Tension also accumulates in the lumbar and sacroiliac regions, giving rise to lumbago and disc herniation. Tightness in the lumbar region has the consequence of loss of tone in the lower abdomen. Consequently, the lower abdomen protrudes and gives rise to a pot belly. Interestingly, Western medicine uses abdominal-to-pelvic girth measurements as predictors of mortality (fig. 2.1).

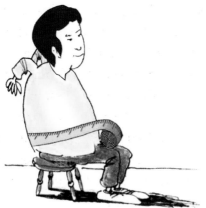

Fig. 2.1. The ratio of abdominal girth to pelvic girth predicts mortality.

Tai Chi creates the correct goals of posture by emphasizing the straight cervical spine, the rounded scapulae, the dropped shoulders, the lumbar spine back, the abdomen in, and the relaxation of the pelvic girdle and hip muscles allowing opening of the kua. This is done by opening awareness to chi. By then making connections to chi and teaching the mind how to receive it, the student can fill the body with chi and consequently remove chronic conditions.

CHOOSING A TAI CHI STYLE

Students may pursue a particular style of Tai Chi because they are attracted to the movements or the philosophy, or simply because they like the teacher. A student might choose the Wu style, for example, because of its lithe movements—like someone choosing a particular form of dance. Or they may appreciate its focus on the internal training of chi and jin. The Wu style's higher stances and small frame may suit those who have not trained in the martial arts, as well as those who are elderly or have medical problems. At the other end of the scale, the option of progressing to a cohesive system of Push Hands and a full-contact boxing system may be a real attraction for some. Some practitioners may wish to add another style to their repertoire, expanding their exploration of Tai Chi.

More often than not, however, the choice of a style of Tai Chi Chuan is based less on the appeal of the style itself than it is on the availability and character of the teacher. It is important to choose a teacher who has a deep knowledge of the art and the ability to meet your needs. The teacher should be ethical, compassionate, and understanding, and should have an eagerness to help others less skilled. Each student's needs will change as she progresses in the art, so it is best to look at the senior students and imagine what it would be like to be in their shoes.

The teacher is both a mentor and guide on the way of the Tao. However, don't get too intense about your selection; you can certainly choose another teacher further down the track, though you will then have to start a new relationship all over again.

The table below highlights some of the key features of the four major Tai Chi styles: Chen, Yang, Wu, and Sun. The Hao style, while a legitimate style, is so rarely seen in the West that it was not included here. (Remember that the Hao style can be called the Wu style as well. However, that *Wu* is pronounced with a falling-rising tone, whereas in the Wu proper style, the name is pronounced with a neutral tone.)

The table below reveals the age of each style based on the life of the founder. In terms of popularity, the Yang style is the most popular, having the biggest number of schools and the richest literature expounding its principles. The second most popular would be the Wu style. The Chen style is less popular perhaps because of the skill required. The Sun style is still emerging, especially in the elderly population.

TAI CHI CHI KUNG STYLES

STYLE	FOUNDER	FLAVOR	FRAME & STANCES	IDEAL PARTICIPANTS
Chen	Chen Wang-Ting (1628–1736)	Mixture of fast and slow, complex martial moves, displays Fa Jin, like a stormy night	Large frame with low stances	Young, martial art experience
Yang	Yang Lu-Chan (1799–1872)	Even pace, flamboyant style, like a flowing river	Large frame most commonly taught	Youth to middle age, no experience necessary
Wu	Wu Chuan-Yu (1834–1902)	Even paced, soft and internal, lithe or snake-like flavor; better suited to contact boxing	Small frame with slanted spine	Suits martial artists interested in boxing; middle-aged and elderly can do form
Sun	Sun Lu-Tang (1861–1931)	Even paced, soft and internal, feminine and Immortal-like	Small frame	Suits elderly or students with medical problems

The Chen style is a complex powerful style that has an outwardly changing tempo. However, beneath this changing tempo there is a deep jin-level consistency. Working with jin is like working a sticky essence in the body and lower tan tien. There is a steady rhythm and a need to pace oneself—much like working with a mortar and pestle. The pops and crackles that signify a release of fa jin are secondary to the inner work and don't interfere with this rhythm. To this point Paul Lam says:

> Essentially, the control of your movements at a more advanced level can be viewed as the evenness of the speed rather than at the same speed. In Chen style, fast and slow are intermixed. The force delivering movements (Fa jin) requires speed. But even in this style, there is evenness within all the variations of the speeds. This evenness contained within different speeds is the key to cultivating elasticity and internal power of your force. In Yang and Sun styles, most of the movements appear to be at the same speed, but with close examination you can find almost unperceivable differences between parts of the movements.[7]

The Chen style's foot stamping and overt displays of Fa Jin make it quite a spectacle. It is like a powerful storm—hard rain and wind punctuated by peals of lightning and thunder. It includes a very low Horse stance that works the kua intensely. Accomplishing this low stance is less difficult for students who started martial arts when young.

Because the display of Fa Jin in the form is a real attraction, we may wonder why Yang Lu-Chan removed Fa Jin from the long form. Most likely he did so because the repetitive and frequent use of Fa Jin can drain jin and deplete the student. Hence this style would exclude the weak and the elderly.

The Yang style was born from the Chen style. It still has the wide-open stances and vertical spine of the Chen style, and there is still the same outward martial display that keeps the postures large and expansive (fig. 2.2). The style is now guided by the principle of water flowing down a gentle stream. Each form has no defined beginning or end and is connected to those before it and after it like running water. A portion of the stream may seem to pause or pool for a moment, but it will continue to spiral and find its way downstream into its next manifestation. This continuous nature gives rise to barely perceptible variations in speed. It evokes Chang San-Feng's principle that "Tai Chi Chuan is like a great river rolling on unceasingly."[8] Therefore, the Yang style can be regarded as an attempt to return to the founder's original purpose. Because it is simpler skill-wise, the form enables the practitioner to really sink and relax into the structure and discover the secrets of moving chi and jin.

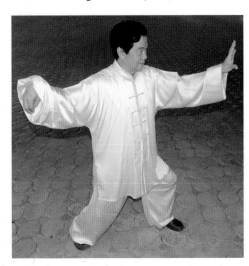

Fig. 2.2. Yang style Single Whip posture

The Wu style evolved from the Yang style and continues to carry its essence, but with some modifications. The Wu style attempts to return to the foundation principles of Tai Chi. Wu Gong-Tsao comments on the Wu style's consistency with Taoism's principles as follows:

> Its movements are light, agile, round, and alive. Therefore, once one moves there is nothing without movement, once one calms there is nothing without calmness. Its theory of movements and calmness is consistent with the sitting *gong* (meditation) of the Dao's family (Daoism).[9]

The Wu masters found that the large frame, vertical spine, and low stances of the Yang are an impediment to the flow of chi and jin (fig. 2.3). By focusing more internally and de-emphasizing external flamboyance, there is more opportunity for internal growth. This internal growth includes elongation of the tendons, which are free to grow as the body fills with chi, the muscle fibers relax, and the limbs lengthen. In other words, by removing blockages and stiffness, the limbs can return to their natural length.

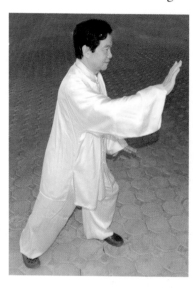

Fig. 2.3. Wu style Brush Knee posture

The overall feeling of the form changes somewhat as it takes on a less outwardly martial outlook and begins to assume the lithesome motion of a snake. This new style avoids interruptions from blockages of chi and jin, and finds grace in coiling, winding, and remaining very connected with the earth.

Perhaps the return to a more functional posture has enabled the style to realign itself with its pugilistic origins and embrace contact boxing once again. The Southern Wu style features a cohesive boxing system, which will be elaborated in chapter 8. A prospective student may be interested in the Wu style because it includes a viable system of self-defense.

The Sun style is two generations away from the Yang style. Sun Lu-Tang learned from Hao Wei-Chen (Hao style) (1849–1920), who studied with Li Yi-Yu (1833–1892), while Li Yi-Yu was a disciple of Wu Yu-Hsiang (1812–1890). Wu Yu-Hsiang studied under Yang Lu-Chan. The Sun style maintains the short and high stances of the small Yang frame (like the Wu style) but includes some synthesized forms from the Bagua and Hsing Yi systems (fig. 2.4). This is in part representative of its founder Sun Lu-Tang, who was also proficient in these internal martial arts.

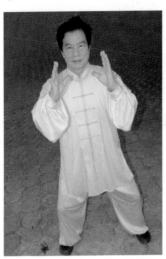

Fig. 2.4. Sun style Closing Hand posture

The Sun forms move with a feminine and even Immortal-like grace, yet still gather power from the tan tien and the earth. The style breaks up the linear progression of forms displayed in the long traditional Yang form and incorporates forms that face the four directions. The four directions herald a return to shamanic traditions that gather the power of the earth, its elements, and the four directions.

In his book *Study of Taiji Boxing*, Sun Lu-Tang states that his form of Tai Chi is a means of improving health;[10] it incorporates the body strengthening aspects of Bagua and Hsing Yi, and also includes Chi Kung. Its Chi Kung elements were added as a vehicle for hastening the acquisition of Postnatal Chi.*

---

*In traditional Chinese medical theory, one's health is determined by the combination of Prenatal Chi (one's genes and health of parents when conceived) and Postnatal Chi. Postnatal life force can be sustained by reducing energetic losses (like excessive menses or ejaculation, poor sleep, inadequate rest, and emotional imbalance) and can be increased by good food and Chi Kung. These aspects will be discussed in chapter 9 of this book.

The Sun style has consequently developed a reputation for being a suitable practice for elderly students or those with medical problems. However, the Yang, Wu, and Sun styles are all applicable to this age sector.

Learning the Southern Wu Style

In the Southern Wu system, the steps and sequence of accomplishment can include the long form, technical Chi Kung exercises (yin and yang), Push Hands, boxing, and weapons. The first step is learning the long square form. For many readers, this will involve learning the shorter sequence taught in this book. The second stage is to learn the round form, which is the square form with the addition of multiple small flowing circles. These small flowing circles are much like the silk-reeling exercises seen in the Chen style and like the parry circles in the Universal Healing Tao Discharge Form. These circular moves are forms within themselves, as well as serving as transitions between forms.

After the square and round forms, a student of the Southern Wu style may learn Chi Kung and technical exercises; these are divided into yin and yang forms. The yin exercises are quiet; they cultivate opening the internal channels and developing the lower tan tien. They correlate with Universal Healing Tao exercises like Embracing the Tree, Holding the Golden Urn, the Golden Turtle, the Buffalo, and the Golden Phoenix Washes Its Feathers.* The yin techniques are also similar to many of the Tan Tien Chi Kung exercises in the Universal Healing Tao system, including the Jade Rabbit, the Dragon, Rhinoceros, and the Bull (Pushing the Sampan Oars).† All of these exercises are intended to fully develop the Iron Shirt, which may ultimately be tested by punches or even by a colleague jumping onto the abdomen.

---

*See Mantak Chia, *Iron Shirt Chi Kung* (Rochester, Vt.: Destiny Books, 2006).
†See Mantak Chia, *Tan Tien Chi Kung* (Rochester, Vt.: Destiny Books, 2004). See also Mantak Chia and Andrew Jan, *Tai Chi Fa Jin* (Rochester, Vt.: Destiny Books, 2012).

The yang forms of Chi Kung are more focused on the power necessary for strikes and blocks within the boxing repertoire. These included the Swallow, Chopping Wood, the Elephant, Leading the Goat, Backward Striking, Civet Cat Catches the Rat, and Flicking Fingers.*

Push Hands can be learned as a skill in and of itself, but it is also a framework on which the principles of boxing can be based. The full-contact fighting system includes segments of the long form performed in real-time speed. Weapons are the final step in the Southern Wu system and include sword, cutlass, and spear. Meditation is not included in this program.

The Universal Healing Tao System and the Southern Wu Style

The Universal Healing Tao system includes much that is similar to the Southern Wu style system described above. Although it does not currently progress to a full-contact fighting system, it can provide a head start for a practitioner wishing to learn the Wu system, or it can provide a complimentary training schedule to enhance a student's training program.

The Universal Healing Tao system also provides a deep and thorough internal training that is lacking in many other styles. The subtle teachings of chi and jin may not have been mastered by all teachers of all styles, or the teachers may follow traditions in which the esoteric aspects of jin are taught only to very select students. In either case, students of many other styles will not be exposed to the skills for developing the internal arts. While the possibility does exist for this power to be used for wrongdoing, for the greater majority it opens a whole new dimension that can lead to healing and ultimately to realization of the Tao.

---

*See Mantak Chia and Andrew Jan, *Tai Chi Fa Jin* (Rochester, Vt.: Destiny Books, 2012).

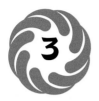

Wu Style Principles

This chapter includes an exploration of:

- Relaxation (*fa song*) and the movement of chi and jin, which are core aspects of Tai Chi that are applicable to the slow form, fast form, Push Hands, and boxing. These will be discussed from the perspective of Iron Shirt principles.
- The issuing of energy including the eight phases and eight gates.
- The basic set of postures and stances used in the Wu form, and differences between it and the Yang style.
- Comments from the founder Chang San-Feng and the various Wu masters: Wang Pei-Shang, Wu-Gong-Tsao, Ma Yueh-Liang, Wen Zee, and Wu Tu-Nan (1884–1987).

FOUNDATIONAL PRINCIPLES

Many fundamental principles are shared by the four major Tai Chi styles. However, because each new style developed as an effort to improve over the previous styles, there are notable differences in how these principles are expressed.

In the Wu style, all postures, movements, and attitudes eventually must conform to the free flow of chi and jin. Wu Gong-Tsao tells us that all forms "will be relaxed, alive, and steady naturally."[1] The movement of chi is associated with such aspects as lightness, calmness, letting go, and the spiritual. Jin, like bread dough, has its own tempo and peculiarities. Jin and chi mutually interact, overlap, and support each other. The concepts that govern chi and jin vary from the Newtonian laws that govern the material plane. The purpose of this chapter is to attempt to describe these concepts. Undoubtedly the reader well knows how intangible some of these are.

The Iron Shirt

The exploration of chi and jin begins with the static postures and the principles of Iron Shirt. One of the beauties of the Universal Healing Tao style is the simple way that it teaches the Iron Shirt. Much of the mystique has been removed to unveil a natural body structure that is conducive to chi flow in all the major meridians with a focus on the Governing and Conception vessels. The consequence of improved flow in the meridians is improved chi flow and functioning of the organs. This, in turn, leads to better health and the realization of the power, strength, and coordination associated with it. Strength is attained because the muscles are elongated to their ideal length and performance characteristics. It is called the Iron Shirt because it makes the chest and abdomen resistant to direct blows.

Because the structure is opened and aligned, the chi and jin can easily flow. Poor coordination is associated with blocked channels, while open channels allow fine coordination. For example, even the simple warm-ups of ankle and wrist rotations become awkward when the lower leg or wrist channels are blocked. This leads to broken and uncoordinated moves during the performance of the complex slow form, and jin cannot pass through the structure. There is no quick or easy way to fill the body with chi. Rather, the cultivation of chi is a combined endeavor of the body, mind, and spirit, encompassing almost every aspect of our daily living, including what and how we eat, our house and living environment, work, friendships, rest, and sleep. But the cultivation of chi mainly resides in practice, which should theoretically be the center of our existence. The student's practice is centered on sitting meditation and expands through standing and moving practice. In sitting practice, learning to relax and become yin is often the biggest lesson. Becoming yin means learning to receive energy from heaven and earth and to align with these forces. This mastery can take a whole lifetime of dedication.

Fa Song

What is required to progress in Iron Shirt training is *fa song. Song* is usually literally translated as "relaxation" and *fa* means "to issue or release." *Fa song* is not as easy as it may sound, however: it is not just becoming limp like a dead fish. The Chinese term for being limp is *ruan; song* is about creating a scaffold or structure first and then relaxing and sinking into the middle of it so that the body can fill with chi. Note, however, that the whole body cannot be too stiff, either. Wu master Wang Pei-Sheng says, "the body should be kept naturally relaxed but not slackened."[2]

What we really want is for the body to be filled with chi and the acupuncture channels to be open. The channels will gradually open with mindful persistence. Some teachers may encourage their students with directions like "be hard on the outside and soft on the inside," or "feel like steel wrapped in cotton wool." It might be clearer if they told their students to "fill the body with chi." Remember, "wherever the mind goes the chi will follow."[3]

In the Microcosmic Orbit meditation the mind should sink and be 95 percent focused on the lower tan tien. This activates the chi and jin which rise up and inflate the structure (see fig. 3.1 on page 30). Wang says, "abide by the Dantian, thus making the whole body vitalized and keeping one's center of gravity lowered and vitalized."[4] What Wang means by "vitalized" is an inflated whole body structure. This force, which arises from sinking or falling into oneself, is what creates the internal power (jin).

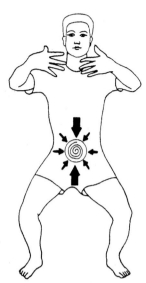

Fig. 3.1. Fill the body with chi by focusing on the lower tan tien.

The term *song* has a flash of serendipity in its pinyin pronunciation, which sounds like the English word *song*. We really want the body to sing rather than just relax. When the body sings it fills the body and channels with chi much more than it could if we were simply to become limp!

How can the student do this? The secret lies in the Fusion meditations that teach us to turn the senses inward. After turning the senses of sight and touch inward, we begin to turn in the sense of hearing (fig. 3.2). This may begin with a high-pitched sound—the "*Eee*" or "*Yang*" sound of the legendary Green Dragon from the East. As you sink deeper into the tan tien, you can hear the "*Ooom*" sound, the yin sound of the immortal White Tiger from the West. The body then reveals a cacophony of sounds in between these two poles that correlate to each of the bones in the body. Eventually the whole body sings and dances to its own tune. This is another way of vitalizing the body and opening the chi channels.*

Once the body can receive and fill itself with chi, its structure begins to change. This process is described in a repetitive mantra that

---

*For more information about turning the senses inward, see *Fusion of the Five Elements* (Rochester, Vt.: Destiny Books, 2007), 52.

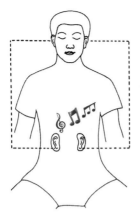

Fig. 3.2. Turning the sense of hearing inward to hear the inner song and help fill the body with chi

the Universal Healing Tao has been reciting to its students for forty years: "The legs externally rotate and lengthen. The kua opens and the coccyx tucks in. The abdomen sucks in, chi goes to the lower tan tien, and the lumbar spine goes back. The scapulae round and the sternum sinks. The arms lengthen and the fingers go soft. The neck lengthens and the chin tucks in" (fig. 3.3).

Wu master Ma Yueh-Liang's student Dr. Wen Zee has a similar

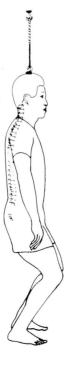

Fig. 3.3. Iron Shirt posture with lifted head

mantra to remind students of these posture changes. The mantra goes: Hui Lin Din Jin ("lift the head and straighten the neck") and Hang Shung Ba Bei ("raise the back and empty the chest").[5]

One of the basic themes of the Iron Shirt posture is the effort to become more yin. This is a difficult endeavor for most people and somewhat contradictory to our Western culture. Just as Western culture can be characterized by the "art of doing," Taoism can be summed up as the "art of doing nothing." Becoming more yin means doing nothing and being patient enough for nature's forces to take over. A good term to describe this process is *apophasis.*

The apophatic principle presumes that Iron Shirt is innate. It is a way of holding the body that we were born with but gradually lose as we learn to compromise our natural state for the sake of survival and socialization. Such compromises and unresolved experiences then create knots and blockages in the body. Some would regard these knots and tensions as an accumulation of ghosts. Ghosts, in Taoist thought, are manufactured by negative emotions such as repressed fear, anger, worries, and sadness. To exorcise attached ghosts that restrict our innate power, the practitioner must consciously remove them. This is most often accomplished through ritual, which can involve the use of talismans, mudras, or simply dedicated Universal Healing Tao practice. Detailed discussion of these rituals is beyond the scope of this text.

Iron Shirt involves undoing the knots and blockages that have accumulated over the years. This is a return to the uncarved block or the state of pu. Pu is achieved by removing tension in the spine, pelvis, and shoulder girdle. In the state of pu we become like children again, receptive to the natural forces around us. The Taoists describe these as heavenly, earthly, and cosmic forces; they strengthen our postnatal chi, open our channels, and revitalize us.

Movement of Chi

Once the structure is relatively organized by the Iron Shirt, chi can be used to mobilize the body for use in Tai Chi forms, Push Hands, or boxing. Chi leads the arms and legs in both closing and opening. It opens the channels and returns the body to the Iron Shirt posture for the smooth passage of jin.

Chi leads the way by opening the channels for the jin. It is cyclical, like the breath (fig. 3.4), beginning—like an exhalation—by closing or contracting the posture and focusing the dispersed jin and yang chi into the lower tan tien and then into the earth. (Dispersed jin can be described as yang chi because it is somewhat prickly and shaky.) Before the jin is released through the body, chi rises up through the legs, spine, and arms, often creating an opening or outward movement of the arms or legs.

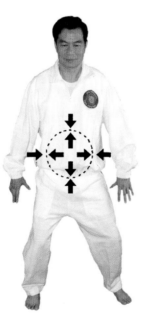

Fig. 3.4. The cyclical nature of chi and jin animates the body via the lower tan tien.

As students become more experienced in Tai Chi practice, they learn to allow chi to move the body, instead of the monkey mind. As in Iron Shirt practice, this involves letting go and becoming aware of the subtle realm of chi. This takes much practice, and as stated above, involves the ability to turn the senses inward. Other helpful things to keep in mind are included below.

The Integrated Mind

In the Universal Healing Tao system, we often quote Yang Chen-Fu, who said, "wherever the mind goes the chi will follow."[6] In this statement, "mind" refers to the three levels of mind that have been integrated into one. The intellectual mind in the upper tan tien becomes the observation mind. The middle tan tien or the heart mind becomes the conscious mind, and the lower tan tien is the awareness mind. All three minds need to settle and merge for the mind to lead the chi.

Another way to understand this integrated mind is to think of the spirit in the upper tan tien, chi in the heart tan tien, and jin in the lower tan tien (fig. 3.5). By staying open and connected to the heavens, the spirit (which can now live in the upper tan tien) has the power to move the chi and in turn the jin. Allowing the spirit to direct the traffic (chi) lets us tap in to something greater. Wu Yu-Hsiang says, "Throughout the body the Yi (mind) relies on the Ching Chen (spirit)."[7]

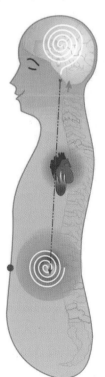

Fig. 3.5. Three minds/ three tan tiens: spirit, chi, and jin

Chi in the Fingertips

Sometimes a simple adjustment of the palms or fingers is all that is needed to get the chi to move the arms or legs. By straightening a finger here or there, the chi can now flow or grasp the limb and move it. In the practice of Chinese medicine, the tips of the fingers and toes include a class of acupuncture points called the Jing Well points (fig. 3.6). Each of these points is located on a particular channel and stimulates its chi flow. The thumb activates the lung channel, the index finger the large intestine channel, the middle finger the pericardium channel, the ring finger the triple warmer channel, and the pinkie finger the heart and small intestine channels. On the foot, the big toe activates the spleen channel, the second toe the stomach channel,

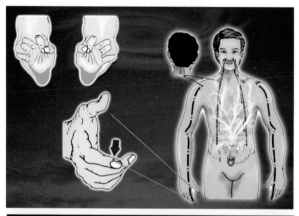

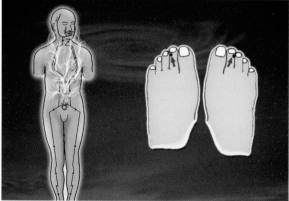

Fig. 3.6. Jing Well and Five Element points
activate the channels and organs.

the fourth toe the gallbladder channel, and the pinkie toe the bladder channel. In Five Element Chi Kung each fingertip activates a different corresponding organ and meridian. The pinkie finger activates the kidney, the ring finger the lungs, the middle finger the heart, the index finger the liver, and the thumb activates the spleen.[8]

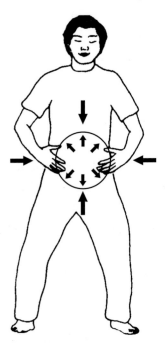

Fig. 3.7. Feeling the subtle connection between the Iron Shirt structure (kua) and the fingertips

When the chi begins to move, it will feel like a subtle and pleasant lightness that opens various parts of the limbs at certain times. This feeling may occur during warm-ups and stretches, which involve continuous subtle movements of the fingers or palms to assist chi flow and the lengthening of the limbs (fig. 3.7). It may also appear during the opening and closing components of Tai Chi moves. In closing moves, use the fingertips to help condense the dispersed jin and yang chi into one point in the lower tan tien. On opening moves—especially before the final Fa Jin release—relax the fingertips more and feel the whole body structure adjust. Slight adjustments of the fingers can result in more tucking of the coccyx, opening of the front kua, and/or opening of the shoulder girdle.

As a student becomes a more experienced practitioner, she will notice additional connections between the fingertips and key components of the Iron Shirt structure. For example, as the hands close to the pelvis, the kua will open. As the hands move past the chest, the sternum sinks. As the hands move toward the head, the third eye opens and the neck becomes long.

Lead with the Large Joints

Another tenet of chi movement is to lead with the large joints and allow the smaller joints to follow. For example, in the opening form of the Wu style, consciously open the armpits slightly. In tandem with adjustment of the fingertips, the arms will automatically rise with chi. The shoulder leads the elbow, which in turn leads the wrist and palm. This is in contrast to the use of li power, where the hand leads the elbow, which leads the shoulder. The laws that govern limb movement with chi are different from those that rely on the monkey mind.

Letting Chi Be the Master

Sometimes chi will want to take you in a different direction than your intellect wants to go. This is an important rite of passage: you think the move should be done this way, but the chi won't move you that way. This can often happen in a class with an overcontrolling instructor, who gives minute instructions about where to place your arm, your foot, your knee, your head, etc. At first, your intellect will obey this voice rather than letting the chi follow its own path. As you progress, the chi becomes the master rather than the voice of a teacher or book. You will learn to follow the chi and see where it takes your body.

Accessing the Spirit

Most Tai Chi moves have lovely metaphors or spirits that shape them. Learn to mimic the white crane, the roc bird, or the action of a whip. The spirit of the posture will help enact the form and connect with the chi.

The Movement of Jin

The difference between jin and chi is a subtle but definite one that is not really discussed much in the classics. Where chi opens the channels, releases tension, and makes minor adjustments without full engagement of muscle groups, jin promotes movement that fully engages the musculoskeletal system and is the basis of true power. Wu master Dr. Zen Wee says that Tai Chi practitioners use the word *jin* to distinguish this power from the monkey mind's muscular power, known as *li* power.[9] Li power does not need chi, whereas jin does. Chi creates a template for the jin to move.

The movement of jin has a cyclical pattern. After Fa Jin, dispersed jin (or yang chi) is gathered into the lower tan tien and then projected down into the earth. This process is called Xu Jin.[10]

DISCHARGING ENERGY: FA JIN

The movement of jin up from the earth into the opponent is called Fa Jin. As jin arises from the earth, it is associated with yin chi and is initially pleasant and smooth. The chi and jin inflate the body structure, including the lower tan tien, which blows out like a balloon just prior to discharge, when the jin can no longer be contained. When the practitioner can't stand the intensity of feeling anymore, he shakes or rotates the tan tien and issues the jin through the chi-primed structure.*

The nature of the release will depend on the gate used and the quality of jin produced in the body. For example, in the two-handed An push, the jin will take on an essence of water or tidal power.

In the slow Wu form—unlike in the fast form, Push Hands, or boxing—the jin is not discharged or ejaculated. Instead, the chi and jin are mainly conserved. In some respects this conservation has similarities with the principles behind Healing Love practice. It is a form of coitus reservatus that keeps the jin contained within the body for

---

*This phase of Fa Jin is analogous to the ejaculation of the pearl through the crown in Fusion and Kan and Li practices.

nourishment and healing. Elderly Chen-style practitioners are advised not to practice Fa Jin too frequently as this can deplete their pre- and postnatal essence. For beginners, it is appropriate that they build up their life force and postnatal essence before embarking on Fa Jin practice. These caveats may help to explain why Yang Lu-Chan and Wu Chuan-Yu kept overt displays of Fa Jin out of the slow form.

In summary, the movement of jin begins by gathering chi and jin into one point in the lower tan tien and into the earth. Chi, soon followed by jin, arises from the earth and prepares the body structure. It fully engages the locomotor system, then, like an orgasm or a burst of madness, it is shivered or ejaculated out of the body.

The Eight Phases of Fa Jin

The eight phases of Fa Jin are components of each Fa Jin release. Each one includes a different posture and different quality of jin in the lower tan tien. Note that the classics and Wu masters have not pieced together the sequence as the authors have done here. Whereas each master highlights several—but not all—of the phases, we have used a syncretic approach to devise this sequence in the hope that it will pull together the teachings of most Tai Chi masters. When only fragments and parts are taught, the student is more likely to fail. Even a detailed presentation like this one is no guarantee of success, however; the final ingredient is always the student's own creative spark within the container of persistent practice.

Phase 1: Sticking to the Opponent or Following the Chi

In the first step of the Xu Jin sequence, the adept needs to develop a sensitivity and softness, so that the body can not only sense the chi but can also be moved by it (see fig. 3.8 on page 41). Wu Gong-Tsao says the adept must be "slow and calm" in order to gain this softness and sensitivity.[11] The chi itself is governed by the interaction of the forces of heaven, earth, and the cosmos.

In Push Hands, this sticking to the opponent is called ting jin. It is part of the mantra of connecting, sticking, adhering, and following, which Wang Tsung-Yueh described this way:

> Zhan, Lian, Nian, and Sui: Zhan is the energy that finds and connects with the partner's energy; Lian is the energy that links and joins with the partner's energy; Nian adheres and merges with the partner's energy; and Sui pursues and follows a partner's energy.[12]

Upon first analysis, zhan, lian, nian, and sui all appear to be the same thing; in fact they are stages in a process of moving from a state of disconnection to a state of merging. In a sparring situation there is no contact: therefore the first aim is to connect (zhan). From there the adept makes an external link with the partner's movement (lian). Going deeper, the adept merges with the partner's internal energetic framework (nian), until finally the merging becomes a unity and it appears that the adept follows (sui) each and every move of the opponent. In actuality they become one.

Listening (ting) uses the language of chi analyzed by the five senses. The monkey mind cannot hear the chi directly—it requires the body and the senses for this. Senses include not only vision and hearing, but also touch, taste, and smell. The first achievement is to turn the mind inward via the five senses, which remain awakened to the body's every move, noticing whether it is grounded or not, fast or slow, light or heavy, connected or disconnected, pushed or pulled. This practice is a fundamental aspect of Fusion of the Five Senses and is perfected in Sealing of the Five Senses. Full understanding—the ability to listen—requires integration of the senses from the upper mind into the body's center—the lower tan tien. Thus we ultimately return to the ideal state, which is our three minds integrated into one. This is where the upper mind (senses), the heart mind (houses the spirit), and the lower mind unite as one force known as the Yi power. Yang Pan-Hou called this level of accomplishment "conscious movement."[13]

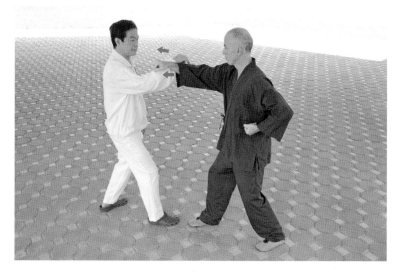

Fig. 3.8. Feel the chi moving the arms.

Phase 2: Formation of Iron Shirt Structure (Drawing the Bow)

Phase 2 correlates to the yin stage of Iron Shirt training wherein an opponent's force is used to open and lengthen the adept's structure.*[14] This collecting (yin) stage could also be described as activating the empty force.[†] This empty force then allows the collection of chi/jin into one point in the lower tan tien (see fig. 3.9 on page 42). It also allows the loading of the bow as the kidneys go back and the coccyx tucks underneath. Wu Yu-Hsiang says, "Store up the chin (internal strength) like drawing a bow."[15] At the same time, keep the entire spine long—including the cervical spine. The creates the sensation of a floating head and space between the base of skull and the occiput. "This is called the suspended head top," says Master Wu.[16]

---

*The classics refer to the Universal Tao's Iron Shirt structure in many ways. In the "Yang Family Forty Chapters," Iron Shirt is referred to as zhong tu ("central equilibrium" or "central earth"). It is also referred to as "standing on the posts" (zhan zhuang) and "in central equilibrium the feet develop root."

†The empty force is the extra power that is generated at the end of exhalation associated with the sucking in of the abdomen.

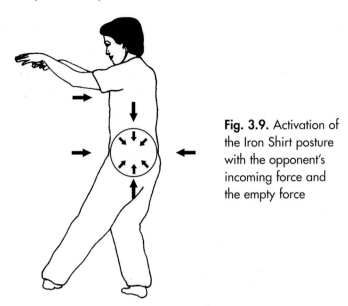

Fig. 3.9. Activation of the Iron Shirt posture with the opponent's incoming force and the empty force

In many respects this yin stage of Fa Jin (known as Xu Jin) is just an extension of Iron Shirt training and pushing. The incoming force is borrowed and utilized to lengthen the spine, open channels, and connect with the empty force. Often, but not always, the breath is emptied and ceases for a brief moment.

In Push Hands and fighting, sticking to the opponent develops sensitivity. The senses are acute and one gains insight into the opponent's intention and balance. In terms of Xu Jin, the force from the opponent is followed, then borrowed and placed in the lower tan tien. It is hard to put such an experience into words. When the novice first learns to take a push, he considers himself to be separate and strong. Later, he realizes that he needs to enjoy the push—as if someone is helping him to stretch inwardly or even giving him a strong therapeutic massage. The key lies in the intention of receiving.

In some respects this dynamic represents the union of two people: it is about merging into one (fig. 3.10). In this sense, the practice has some similarities to Bedroom Kung Fu and Healing Love—teaching the student how to receive and merge. Chang San-Feng supports this notion of merging through jin in the thirty-ninth chapter of Yang Pan-Hou's Forty Chapters. He explains that this receiving is more powerful than single cultivation of sexual energy. He says, "to seize the female within our own bodies is not as good as the interaction of yin and yang between two males, for this is a more rapid method of self-cultivation."[17]

In other words, borrow the jin from your Push Hands opponent (or from the forces of heaven, earth, and cosmos if you're practicing alone) and bring it into the tan tien in order to strengthen yourself. To do this, have the intention of nourishment and support rather than fear, separateness, or a desire to win.

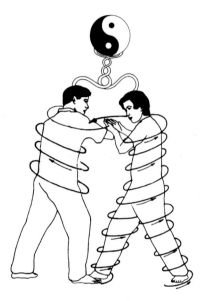

Fig. 3.10. Two practitioners connecting with chi and becoming one

Phase 3: Transformation

The phase of transformation exemplifies the mystique and magic of discharge power. In this phase, forces are taken to a stillpoint deep in the earth and the lower tan tien, and there they are transformed. The student sinks within and lets go of all the holding patterns that have previously denied access to this power. He trusts that he will not fall, and that the chi and jin will not only hold him up but will also supply a new untold power (see fig. 3.11 on page 44).

In Push Hands, the collection of jin and connection to the earth are used to a further advantage. They give both heaviness and buoyancy, which are required to meet the chaotic and unpredictable demands of

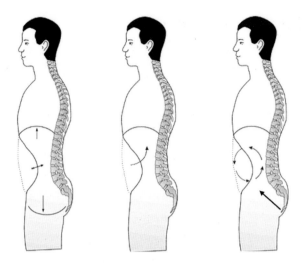

Fig. 3.11. Acitivation of the structure
with the empty force

free Push Hands. Wu Gong-Tsao offers the terrific metaphor of a toy tumbler—a child's weighted toy that always returns to a standing position, even after being knocked down (fig. 3.12). He suggests that this toy can guide the way the students hold themselves, keeping heaviness in the lower tan tien and the earth while maintaining lightness in the arms.[18] No matter how disturbed the arms may get, the chi and jin continue to be drawn to the lower tan tien and earth, which creates a low sense of gravity and rootedness. Furthermore, the harder you hit a toy tumbler the more the toy swings back at you.

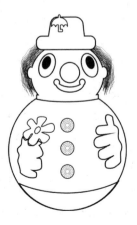

Fig. 3.12. Toy tumbler

Phase 4: Rotation and Taking Aim

While power is still in its undifferentiated or quiescent form, the adept can begin to prepare to move the jin in the chosen direction. This is more easily achieved if she has opened the Central Thrusting Channel (Chong Mai). The body can rotate around the Thrusting Channel while maintaining the Iron Shirt structure (fig. 3.13).

The Central Thrusting Channel comes into play in the central and forward positions and also enables power to be released left or right. The importance of the mind and waist rotation in the execution of discharge power is highlighted by Yang Pan-Hou when he says, "With one wave of the signal flag the wheels of the two Ming Men begin to turn. When orders are issued by the mind, the chi goes into action like army banners."[19]

The rotation of the waist can vary from small to large. For example, in a straight two-hand Push the circle can be minimal, whereas with the Lieh force, it is likely to be more pronounced.

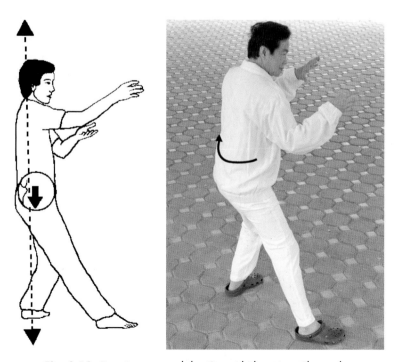

Fig. 3.13. Rotation around the Central Thrusting Channel

Phase 5: Chi and Jin Appear from the Earth

From stillness an initial force appears. This initial force prepares the root in the legs, sacrum, and waist and is the foundation for the ultimate release of Fa Jin (fig. 3.14). This foundation loosens the structure and creates a milieu for the spark or Big Bang to appear.

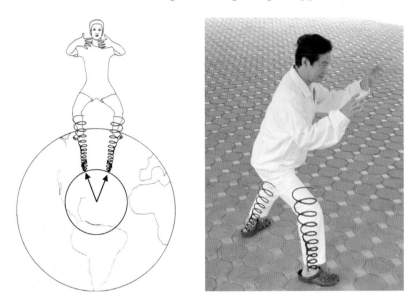

Fig. 3.14. Primordial Chi coming from the earth

Phase 6: Expansion of the Lower Tan Tien

The rush of chi appears to come from the earth and pass up through the legs to the lower tan tien. The kidneys separate from the navel. For a moment, the chi/jin is stored in the lower tan tien (fig. 3.15). The quality of energy in the lower tan tien will vary according to the gate or force that will be required. (See page 51 for more information about these gates.)

Phase 7: Passage of Chi/Jin Through the Structure While Preparing Application

This facet of Fa Jin is practiced in Tai Chi Chi Kung training, where the power from the earth is released in an effortless and structured manner. In phase 3, power received by the opponent is stored in the earth and

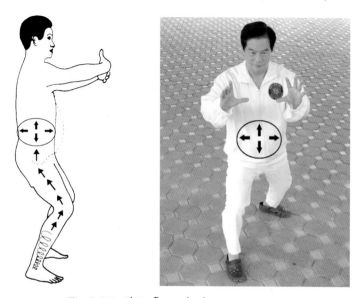

Fig. 3.15. Chi inflates the lower tan tien.

the lower tan tien. In this phase, that power is released through the body in a specific pattern. The jin or power ascends from the feet via the legs, which are kept in their rooted form. Wu Gong-Tsao says, "The root is at the feet generated from the legs, mastered by the waist, and manifested at the fingers."[20] The legs are lengthened because the coccyx is tucked under and the front kua is opened. Power is released via the entire spine (see fig. 3.16 on page 48). "Strength is issued from the spine," says Wu Yu-Hsiang.[21] The arms are connected to the power via C7 and the rounded scapulae. If the adept has a broken structure then the final jin force cannot be discharged freely. To this point, Chang San-Feng says, "all parts of the body must be light, nimble, and strung together."[22]

It is important that chi lead the way through the structure just prior to the jin rising. This means that the body and the distal extremities must remain soft, loose, and relaxed. The chi will then keep the limbs lengthened so that the jin can pass unimpeded to the fingertips.

The whole structure is now prepared for the final climax. It is fully bathed in Primordial Chi awaiting the final spark. The opponent is also now at the zenith of imbalance. Four ounces is now all that is needed to throw the victim.

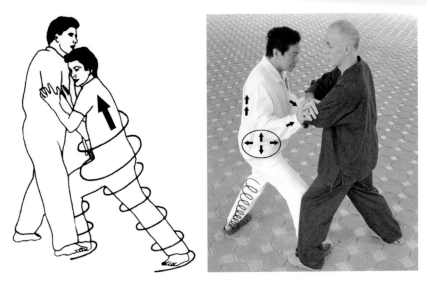

Fig. 3.16. Chi/jin moving up the body and spine

Phase 8: Discharge of Power into the Opponent*

The Big Bang can now occur, and then we can begin all over again. Yang jin from the opponent is courted by the yin of the adept into stillness or nothingness in the earth (neutralization). For a moment it expands and then reaches a point of no return; it explodes and is released as discharge power (fig. 3.17). This discharge disperses chi and jin, which then must be gathered for the whole cycle to be repeated. Alternating cycles of Xu Jin and Fa Jin occur ad infinitum, much like the oscillating cyclical contraction and expansion of the universe purported by Taoists and supported by modern physics. The Taoist cosmological doctrine forms the basis of Tai Chi and thus validates it as a path toward immortality.

The shaking of the jin that occurs in this phase can be extremely dangerous and has the potential to dislocate joints or break bones. It should be used with caution, and it is restricted for older practitioners as it can drain postnatal essence.

The discharge of power occurs not because the adept wills it, but

---

*Please note that in the slow form, only phases 1–7 are used. Phase 8 is reserved for the fast form, Push Hands, and boxing.

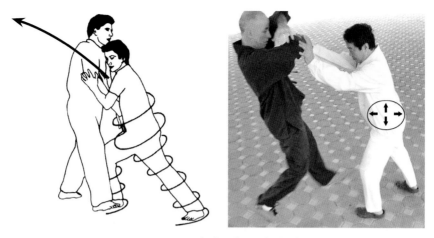

Fig. 3.17. Jin explodes through the body.

because it is unstoppable. This is because the whole body structure remains open, the breath has been held to some degree, and the body sensations are overwhelming. It is in some respects like an orgasm, wherein the jin has been held in the body beyond the point of no return and must release. It is much the same process as occurs in the Fusion and Kan and Li meditations when it is time for the blissful energy to leave via the crown (see fig. 3.18 on page 50). This ejaculation of the energy body out of the physical structure must occur before the adept can form the spiritual body.

Alternatively, practitioners such as Erle Montaigue claim that holding on to the jin reaches a point that feels like a madness. It cannot be contained and so must be released.[23] As the jin has filled the body and reached the point of no return, the body shivers or spirals in the lower back. The adept shakes her back like a dog shaking water off its body. There is now no friction or impedance to this force. The pathway has been laid open by the prior stages, and the body has expanded with Primordial Chi.

The arms are able to transfer this power because the arm tendons rotate in a particular pattern that follows the jin or energy as it travels through the spine. In the standard Two-Hand Push, C7 goes back; the scapulae rotate medially from their inferior portion as well

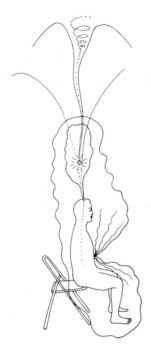

Fig. 3.18. Blissful ejection of energy through the crown in advanced meditation

as spreading out laterally. The elbows drop and the hands laterally rotate. This bending of the elbows and external rotation of the hands are of vital importance. As Wu Yu-Hsiang reminds us, "In the bent seek the straight."[24] We practice this transfer of power through the arms in the Tao Yin postures of Bow and Arrow and Dragon Tucks in its Tail and Stretches its Claws.

Just as the adept's body has been prepared for this final jin, so, too, has the opponent's body. His structure has already been broken, and he is on the point of imbalance. This creates an ideal situation, where four ounces of force is all that is needed. Wang Pei-Sheng's Wu style manual says:

> At the point of issuing energy, your eyes are looking at the direction toward which you are to issue energy, and yourself and your opponent should be linked together into one, so the contacting point should not be shifted at all, and therefore needs no attention . . . the energy you are sending out could then reach the target you have set on your opponent's body instantly.[25]

The Eight Gates

When power is discharged in phase 8, it can manifest along eight different pathways or gates. These are known as Peng, Lu, Ji, An, Tsai, Lieh, Chou, and Kou.

Peng

Peng is the internal energy that results in relaxed resistance within the body. Peng is generated from the original source that inflates the body from the inside. It is like a spring that is ready to be released; the closest element would be wood power.

Lu

Lu cultivates extreme yin and requires a body memory of the Wu Wei or emptiness. For many students, this may start as visualization. With time, the body integrates the knowledge into movement. Therefore, one moves from visualization to actualization.

The magical Lu is able to lead an opponent's force into a desired direction. It is magical because it typifies the transformative power of softness in martial arts and because it is in itself a gateway to all the other gates.

Ji

The Ji force is characteristically performed using the Press from the Bird's Tail form but can be used in any other movement. This discharge force is like a coin bouncing off a drum. The tan tien expands and stretches the fasciae of the body like the skin of a drum or the strings of a tennis racquet; the opponent is then bounced away with seemingly minimal effort. Releasing the power of the Ji force is more effective when the opponent is on the brink of toppling over.

An

According to Tan Meng-Hsien, the principle of this discharge is water. Through careful listening by the practitioner, every small crevice or break in the opponent's structure is filled with water chi. Through the effortless power of water, the opponent is backed up until he has no reserve. His structure is broken and a only a feather is now needed to move him.

Lieh

The internal manifestation of this force is a spinning disc or whirlpool. This sensation is created in the tan tien and extends around the Central Thrusting Channel. Any external force that enters the body wayward of the center will be caught up in the centrifugal force and be cast out faster than it entered. Therefore, to cultivate this force the central axis or axle must be internally defined through sitting practice and standing meditation.

The external manifestation of this movement originates with both arms starting their journey close together, but vectors of force can fly from the center at varying angles, thus enabling the power of a double strike.

Tsai

This force is characterized by leverage—usually at the elbow, but it can easily be applied to the wrist, shoulder, or torso. Tsai takes over from the Lu force, which lengthens the opponent's arm to break his Iron Shirt structure. The Tsai force then locks the elbow and uses it as leverage to either take the opponent to the ground or fling him off.

Chou

The Chou force uses the elbow as an alternative striking implement to the hands. There are times when the hand is still engaged and the opponent is within short striking distance; in this case, the elbow can be used. The inner manifestation of the Chou force is described by Tan Meng-Hsien as maintaining within the body the varied energies of yin and yang (full and empty), and the five elements.

Kou

Kou—the Shoulder Strike—can be used in various situations, from an unsuspecting neutral position to a last-resort counter attack similar to the one described above with the elbow strike. The Kou force's internal energetic image is that of a pounding pestle. This release of power relies on creating a strong Iron Shirt structure via connection with the opponent.

PRINCIPLES AND GUIDANCE FOR DEVELOPING THE WU SLOW FORM

A student of the Wu style slow form must first discover the principles that are universal to all the styles of Tai Chi: the teachings of Chang San-Feng, Wang Tsung-Yueh, Wu Yu Hsiang, Yang Pan-Hou, and Li Yi-Yu are important initial steps in this regard. We also recommend the excellent translation and commentary on Wu Gong-Tsao's "Lecture of Taijiquan" by Dr. Yang Jwing-Ming. Specific Wu style texts include the teachings of masters Wang Pei-Sheng, Ma Yueh-Liang, Wen Zee, and Lee Tin-Chan. All of these are included in the bibliography at the end of this text.

When exploring the Wu style in particular, we begin with the basic postures and the Iron Shirt principles embedded in them. Next, we learn how to link the postures to each other using the movement of chi and jin and the principles of substantial and insubstantial (Xu Jin and Fa Jin).

Beneath the cyclical nature of chi and jin there is the nothingness of the void—the calmness and stillness that the great masters have forever been reminding us of. This is the constancy that paradoxically connects the postures to the principles of yin and yang throughout the form. Once calm and still, the forms can then be embellished with martial spirit, giving their true meaning that becomes visible as power, vigor, and coordination.

The Basic Postures or Stances

The seven main postures in the Wu style are the Parallel, Treading, Bow, Horse, Sitting Back, One Leg, and Half Split stances.*

Parallel Stance

The Parallel stance (fig. 3.19) is used in the opening and closing forms, Step Forward, and Stand Up.

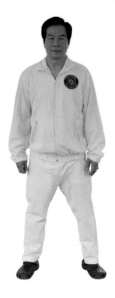

Fig. 3.19. Parallel stance

Bow and Treading Postures

The Bow and Treading postures are variations of the stances used in the Brush Knee and Bird's Tail (fig. 3.20). The Bow is really the standard forward stance used in Tai Chi, but in the Wu style the feet are closer together and more parallel compared with the Yang style. This Bow posture creates some stability in balance, as the martial intention and the opposite leading leg counterbalance momentum of the leading arm. In the Treading posture, the arms are reversed, such that the lead arm is raised over the same side lead leg. This posture occurs in

---

*These are the postures proposed by Lee Tin-Chan in his book, *The Wu Style of Tai Chi Chuan* (Burbank, Calif.: Unique Publications, 1982).

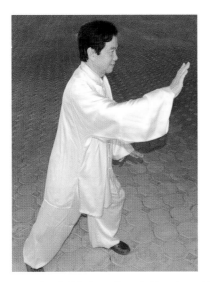
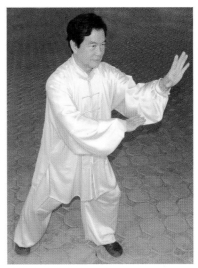

Fig. 3.20. Bow (Brush Knee) and Treading (Slap the Face) postures

the short form in the Bird's Tail and in the long form in forms such as Part the Horse's Mane.

Horse Stance

The Horse stance is almost universal in the martial arts (fig. 3.21). In Iron Shirt practice, we encourage students to use a high stance. This helps the student avoid using li power and become more yin.

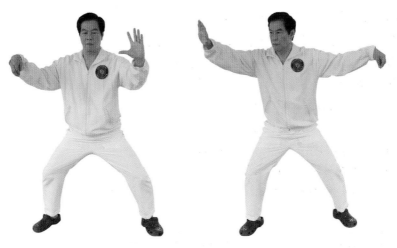

Fig. 3.21. Horse stance and Single Whip

However, for the purpose of the slow form, a lower wider stance should be used. This lower stance engages more of the muscles around the pelvic girdle. It also helps open the kua to a greater degree. The Horse stance is used in the Single Whip and is found in the long form in such postures as Fan through the Back.

Sitting Back

Sitting Back is used in the back position of the Bird's Tail (fig. 3.22). In the long form, it is used overtly in the Seven Star form, and it also occurs in all transitions from forward to back postures. Many students have difficulty with this posture and need to learn to push the Ming Men point back. Moving the Ming Men back requires working the perineum, using the Empty Force, and opening the Microcosmic Orbit. Once the kidneys are back there is stability and power in this posture.

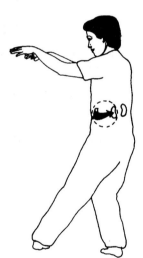

Fig. 3.22. Sitting Back with kidneys back

Half Splitting

The Half Splitting form is where the rear leg is externally rotated and flexed at the knee while the front foot is pointed forward with the knee more extended (fig. 3.23). It requires loosening the adductors and opening the kua. Older practitioners will need to release bracing and holding patterns in the groin. Squatting, the Golden Turtle posture, and Chi Weight Lifting are all useful adjuncts to assist this opening.

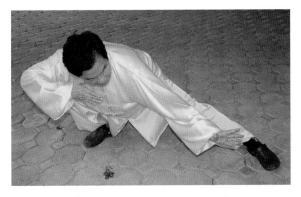

Fig. 3.23. Half Splitting posture in Snake Creeps Down

This posture is not used in the short form, but is found in the long form in Snake Creeps Down.

One Legged

One Legged posture appears in the long form as the Golden Cock Stands on One Leg (fig. 3.24). The ability to perform this posture relies on lightness and the activation of the meridians in the raised leg. Using chi rather than li power, the posture becomes effortless. Ideally, the whole body will feel as if it is floating up, rather than being forced up.

While many of these postures are not included in the Universal

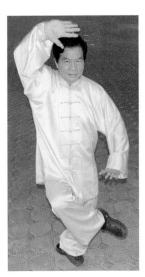

Fig. 3.24. Golden Cock Stands on One Leg

Healing Tao Form, it is still wise for the student to practice them: each posture variant helps to develop different muscle groups and meridians, each meridian has a unique connection to the organs and therefore an effect on body function, and each posture has differences in martial application. These benefits are especially important for those who are near accomplishment of the short form and ready to progress to the long form. Remember that the Iron Shirt principles can be applied to any posture.

The Slanted Spine

As we have earlier discussed, the spine is more slanted in the Wu form than it is in the traditional Yang form. (Remember that the Universal Healing Tao Tai Chi Chi Kung Yang Slow Form and Discharge Form are closer to the Small Yang Frame, and so they already manifest features of the Wu form.) What does the slanted spine imply in terms of Fa Jin and form?

First, the slanted spine allows the passage of jin through the structure more easily than a more vertical spine (fig. 3.25). The reader should take a moment to feel this difference: by tucking in the sacrum, pushing back with the lumbar spine, pushing back the thoracic spine, widening the scapulae, reducing the cervical lordosis, and finally tuck-

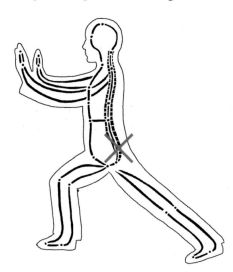

Fig. 3.25. The wide Yang stance shows a blockage of chi at the junction of the pelvis and the lumbar spine.

ing in the chin. You will find that this posture is not only more difficult with a vertical spine, but also that the upper spine moves significantly backward in order to compensate for the vertical spine. It also has a tendency—unless you are very flexible—toward dissociation between the legs and the trunk. Second, the slanted spine enables a downward vector during strikes; this will be discussed below with reference to palm strikes.

Hand Positions and the Palm Strike

In the Northern style of the Wu form, the hands begin the Brush Knee movement with the hand above the shoulder in an initially awkward yet natural position (fig. 3.26). The palm is rotated inward, thumb sitting opposite the third finger, fingers slightly flexed. The metacarpophalangeal joints (connecting the fingers to the palms) are also flexed. The wrist is slightly flexed and deviated toward the ulna. All of this may sound extremely complicated, but it is just a way to achieve a relaxed soft palm in this over-the-shoulder position.

For the purpose of describing movement of the arm, we shall presume that the jin has already passed through the whole body and

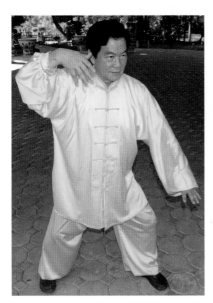

Fig. 3.26. Northern Wu palm for Brush Knee Strike

begun activating the arm. As jin passes through the body it activates the nerves and muscle groups in a natural way. Passing up the spine, it activates the myotomes—muscle groups that correspond to spinal nerves—of T1 through C5. While knowledge of the exact anatomy is not required for execution of the Wu form, it can highlight the following point: as the jin passes through the myotomes via the nerves, it coordinates muscle contraction that is beyond direct control of the monkey mind (fig. 3.27). In other words, let the jin naturally pass up the spine and into the arm—with a slight shaping from the heart mind (Yi)—and the arm will unfold and release its power.

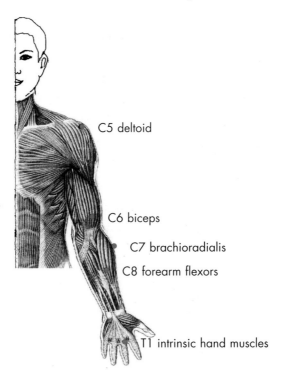

C5 deltoid

C6 biceps

C7 brachioradialis

C8 forearm flexors

T1 intrinsic hand muscles

Fig. 3.27. Arm muscles corresponding with myotomes

In the Northern style, the Brush Knee striking palm is much like a snake striking or a bird landing on water. The Universal Healing Tao Form is consistent with the Southern Wu school and has drifted somewhat back toward the Yang style (fig. 3.28); the hand begins as a flat palm above the shoulder. The hand is still slanted, however, and

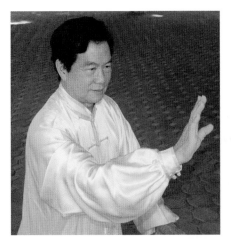
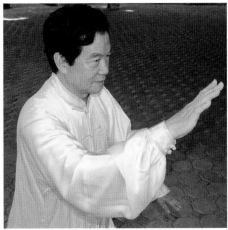

Fig. 3.28. Yang palm and Southern Wu palm

the strike varies with the amount of heel palm strike that is exerted at the last moment of impact.

It is with this particular form of palm strike in Brush Knee that a force arises in the Wu style that is different from the Yang style. Whereas the overall force is more horizontal in the Yang style, the Wu style now adds a downward vector to the palm strike.

The jin is still passed up the body, but at the last minute there is room to accommodate a sinking motion as the palm connects with its (imaginary or real) target. The slanted posture in combination with an angled palm allows the practitioner to strike with a downward vector (fig. 3.29). A slight buckling of the knees and an intended

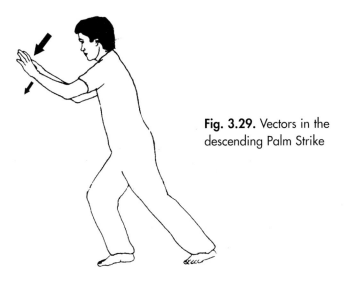

Fig. 3.29. Vectors in the descending Palm Strike

transference of the body weight to the opponent can enhance this downward force. In this strike, power comes up from the ground providing force in a horizontal direction, and the practitioner can also add a descending force. If timed correctly, the practitioner's whole body weight can be transferred to the opponent, creating a most powerful strike.

The slanted spine not only facilitates a downward vector and transfer of body weight in a Palm Strike, but it can also facilitate uprooting. Uprooting using the Kou force with a vertical spine is problematic, but an angled spine enables extended reach before the jin is released. The primary vector can also be released in accordance with the direction of the spine, rather than directly upward as with a vertical spine (fig. 3.30).

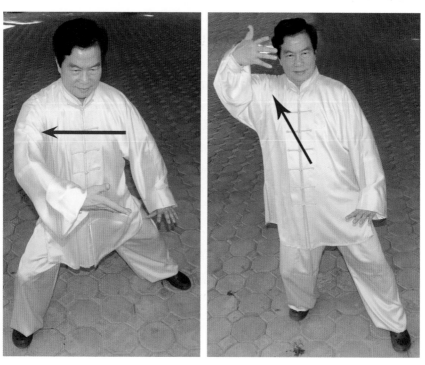

Fig. 3.30. Flying Oblique and vectors in the Yang versus Wu styles

Of course, there is a downside with the slanted spine. There is a potential for overshoot and the uprooting of the practitioner. This could occur if the opponent exerts a Lu force or the practitioner strikes and misses the target. Good listening and understanding (ting and dong) can minimize the risk of overshooting while not preempting the strike.

In the practice of Tai Chi, each realm of our mundane existence and awkward movement must go through the process of being embellished with chi. First the mind must transition from its intellectual ego state into one that integrates chi and the whole body. Second, all postures, movements, and martial forms must also integrate with this life force. The body and mind take on a larger dimension and have to follow its new laws.

Transition from the intellectual monkey mind to an integrated state is the hallmark of progress in Tai Chi. From being scattered and having a totally disorganized body, we master the basic Wu postures with Iron Shirt principles. These postures are then polished into the five moves (forward, backward, left, right, and center) and the eight gates. From this condensation to Thirteen Postures we merge with the trinity of chi, jin, and spirit, which provide continuity between the various postures and forms. From this trinity we reduce experience to a duality of substantial and insubstantial, and then finally we approach the oneness of the Tao.

In this chapter we have explored the fundamental principles that help a student to master the Wu form. There are many processes that must occur simultaneously; this chapter attempted to define the steps and phases whereby the awkward mundane movements of the beginner become accomplished Tai Chi—the supreme Ultimate.

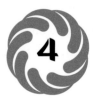

Wu Style Warm-Ups

The aim of this chapter is to describe the goals, methods, and theory behind the warm-ups found in Tai Chi, and in the Wu system in particular. Warm-ups will be described with the intention of accomplishing Tai Chi goals, including the yin and yang techniques used in the Wu style. Some comparisons will be made between the Western scientific understanding of warm-ups versus a Taoist one.

Specific warm-ups are not featured in current mainstream texts for the Wu system. Furthermore, many schools incorrectly proceed immediately into the long form as a warm-up, then practice the form a second time once it has been "warmed up" by the first one. In cases where the boxing or Push Hands are the purpose of the training session, Push Hands is often carried out in a lighthearted manner until the body is warm. Some schools may practice internal techniques as warm-ups prior to the slow form, Push Hands, or boxing. The yin techniques are practiced before the slow form while the yang technicals are best before martial applications.

GOALS OF WARM-UPS

The purpose of warm-ups for Tai Chi has overlap in both content and purpose with Western sports, other martial arts, and the various styles of Tai Chi. From a Western perspective, the purpose of a warm-up is to prepare the body for peak performance in the chosen discipline while simultaneously lowering the likelihood of injury. Technical exercises or drills practice a specific skill that will be used in real-time during the activity.

From a Western perspective, warm-ups literally warm the body and its various tissues, many of which perform most efficiently at warmer temperatures. These include: muscles and nerves, which contract more efficiently in a warmed state; the vital organs such as the heart and lungs, which take in oxygen and deliver it to the tissues more efficiently when warm; and synovial fluid, which reaches an ideal viscosity when warm for cushioning and protecting the joints. Some researchers also acknowledge the role of the mind in warm-ups. Author Robert Kriegal describes a state of mind he calls the "C zone," which is conducive to peak performance and minimizing injury.[1]

Among the different Tai Chi schools, the goals of warm-ups are fairly similar to each other and can be found in the classic texts. As Chang San-Feng, the founder of Tai Chi, says:

> Whenever one moves, the entire body must be light and lively, and must all be connected throughout. The qi should be excited; the spirit should be gathered within. Let there be no hollows or projections; let there be no stops and starts. Its root is in the feet, its issuing from the legs, its control from the yao and its shaping in the fingers. From the feet, to the legs, and then the yao; there must be completely one qi.[2]

Here Chang San-Feng emphasizes that the body, chi (qi), and spirit must be awakened. The "hollows and projections" refer to those parts of the body that are blocked and therefore prevent the formation of the Iron Shirt posture. The yao refers to the waist, including the lower tan tien and the Belt Channel (Dai Mai). "One qi" means that the various energies throughout the body are connected and able to work as one unit.

Three Minds Into One

Wu Gong-Tsao urges us to integrate the three minds and the body. "Feel in the body and awareness in the heart. The body feels, the heart is aware."[3] Integrating the three minds and the body helps make the transition from a body with multiple contractions and chi blockages to a body that is open. It moves the student from a clumsy state to a calm, centered, coordinated one—from a state where the monkey mind reigns with li power to one where the mind and locomotor system have integrated with the life force, so that chi and jin can be used to execute movement.

The following table highlights the differences between the everyday clumsy state and the warmed-up state, which integrates the three tan tiens and the body.

AREA OF BODY	EVERYDAY STATE	WARMED-UP STATE
MIND—upper tan tien	Rooted in thought, in the "monkey mind"	Rooted in the body and connected to the heavens
HEART—middle tan tien	Often closed	Open, spirit awakened. Warmth from the heart radiates through the body.
WAIST—lower tan tien	Closed and tight	Open: lumbar open, sacrum tucked in, connected to the earth. Tan tien awakened, with Belt Channel, Central Thrusting Channel, and Governing and Conception Channels open.
BODY	Low blood flow to joints and muscles. Synovial fluid is sticky, fasciae crinkled, and organ energies are stagnant.	Lively with increased blood flow to joints and muscles; synovial fluid warmed and lubricating while fasciae are comfortably stretched open. Organ energies are balanced.
CHI (acupuncture channels)	Often stagnant with "hollows and protuberances"	Microcosmic Orbit, tan tiens, and Belt channel are all open.

Free Movement of the Arms

When the body and mind have not been properly prepared by warm-ups, a student can only practice at the lowest level of the form, which is akin to the everyday state of mind and the realm of the ten thousand things. The mind is stuck in the head and the body resorts to li power. At the highest level of the form, on the other hand, the limbs appear to float freely and are directed by the chi in the lower tan tien. The chi is sunk such so that the body is mobile with a low center of gravity. Wu Gong-Tsao says, "It is just like a toy tumbler. The top is light and the low is sunk."[4]

This is a useful metaphor to use in the warm-ups and will be described in more detail in the practical section of this chapter. Basically, the arms merely float or move around in response to rotation or movement in the lower tan tien.

Freedom of rotation around the central axis was an important principle taught in the Yang school. Remember Yang Pan-Hou's statement:

> The two arms are like a balance that swings left and right. The waist is the stem of the balance. . . . The plumb line suspending the head and the base of the balance located in the waist connect the Wei Lu point in the coccyx and the Hsin Men point at the crown of the head.[5]

Here, the Central Thrusting Channel that connects the crown to the perineum is the Tai Chi Pole, around which the sides of the body can rotate left or right. The toy tumbler feels like a more apt metaphor, because it not only includes rotation to the left and right, but also allows movement forward and backward. It thus provides an easy image of the stability required to master the five postures. It also incorporates the innovative changes of the Wu style's slanted spine into that image.

The focused chi and jin in the lower structure—analogous to the weight placed in the base of the tumbler—is concordant with the narrower stance of the Wu style. Ma Yueh-Liang says, "There are but two ways to insure the stability of the center of gravity. One is to lower the center of gravity; the other is to enlarge the area of the supporting space."[6] The Wu style seeks stability more through the internal center of gravity than in the large-frame postures. This is another example of its drift toward refinement and focus of the mind. It also ensures that age is no longer a barrier for this art. Wu Chuan-Yu, who was taught by Yang Pan-Hou, seems to have improved the more two-dimensional perspective set out by the Yang school. He debunked the obsessive necessity to have a cumbersome wide-based stance.

The Role of Spirit

The ideal state involves a reduction in experience from the multiplicity found in the mind, which is stuck in the realm of the ten thousand things. Lee Tin-Chan—a student of Southern Wu master Wu Kam-Chin—provides us with a useful way to condense multiplicity into a duality and then into oneness. He says:

> Transform the physical body through motion to generate more life fluid. Transform the life fluid into circulating breath. Combine life fluid and circulating breath with life spirit. Transform life spirit into the void.[7]

The interplay of life, spirit, and the void is an echo of the interplay of the substantial and insubstantial. This complex weaving manifests in the Tai Chi dynamics of opening and closing, sinking and floating, breathing in and breathing out, advancing and retreating, fa jin and xu jin.

THE COMPLETE, INTEGRATED WARM-UP

A good warm-up will accomplish a multiplicity of goals for the body, mind, and spirit. The table below illustrates the many dimensions of an effective Tai Chi warm-up.

THE INTEGRATED WARM-UP

ASPECT OF SELF	EVERYDAY STATE	WARMED-UP STATE
Mind	Monkey mind	Integrated three minds
		Mind collaborates with chi and jin
	Mind scattered	Mind still
Nerves and senses	Senses outward	Body tunes into the "song"
	Body insensitive	Body sensitive to chi
	Non-enjoyment	Pleasure in movement and bodily sensations
Muscles	Muscles tense	Muscles relaxed
	Li power	Jin power
Channels	Blocked	Open
Connection	Disconnect between postures	Connected by chi and jin
	Sense of separateness	Sense of spirit connection to animals, others, etc.
		Connection to stillness via substantial and insubstantial
Breath	Breath high and fast	Breath slow, whole-body breathing
Coordination	High center of gravity	Body sunk and low center of gravity
	Clumsy	Coordinated
	Double-weighted	Movement obeys cyclical laws of substantial and insubstantial

With so many things to accomplish, it can be difficult for practitioners to hone in on the most important components of a warm-up routine. In *Tai Chi Fa Jin*, we listed the characteristics of an ideal warm-up as follows:

- Integrated Mind
- Balanced Organ and Emotional Energy

- Stretching
- Plyometrics/Calisthenics
- Rotations
- Percussion and Shaking

Integrated and Connected Mind

Integrating the three minds and balancing the organs is a foundation practice of the Universal Healing Tao system. Accomplishing this integration within the warm-up is vital for optimum functioning.

The philosophy behind the practice acknowledges that mind is certainly more than the narrow Western perspective, which locates thought, perception, and cognition solely within the confines of the cranium. The integrated mind encompasses these three broad aspects: the observation mind of the brain, the consciousness of the heart, and the awareness of the gut mind.

If the heart is not passionate then there will be no success in any venture. The spirit that connects all living creatures must be awakened; as we understand from Taoist energetic physiology, the spirit (Shen) resides in the heart. The heart must be open to become free.

The gut mind and the lower tan tien have much overlap both anatomically and in terms of functionality. The gut mind creates that primal awareness that is associated with gut instinct. Numerous aphorisms in our culture instruct us not only to follow our hearts; they also frequently refer to the importance of the perception of the intestines. The lower tan tien in the integrated state becomes both the center of awareness and prime mover for ideal coordinated movement and form. It is the weight that provides the magic of the toy tumbler.

Balanced Organ and Emotional Energy

There is an equilibrated state that sits comfortably between yin and yang; this balanced state allows us to access the energies we need in the right measure. The ability to access the yang and yin energies—as well as the spirits of each organ—from a centered state is the key to a coordinated act.

Excessive fear, worry, and anger, etc., are yang energies that create contracture and poor coordination, thereby denying us access to the spirits and yin energies. Being tense and contracted also prevents the release of yang energies in appropriate circumstances. Yang energies include not only the negative emotions but also the energies and spirits of the animals associated with each organ. The Taoist totem includes the ferocious spirit of the dragon, the quickness and precision of an attacking pheasant, the sad and heavy retreat of the beaten tiger, the rapid retreat of the frightened deer, and the alert protective nature of the phoenix.

Yin energies are also required to ensure a balanced form or healthy combat. The yin energies include: the tortoise, whose contraction into a shell is akin to the last-resort Iron Shirt protection; the intelligent listening and adhering energy of the dragon; the penetrating courage of the tiger; the inviting quality of the phoenix; and the connecting and accepting nature of the pheasant.

Of course the armamentarium is not confined to the five totem animals, but can expand to include others from the Wu style: the snake, white crane, golden cock, roc bird, and the monkey are all evoked during the long form.

Stretching

Western sports physiology promotes stretching because it activates the proprioceptors (position-sense nerve endings) and increases range of movement of the joints. Both benefits are vital for neuromuscular coordination and movement.

To Western thinking, stretching involves an act of forced elongation of select muscle groups. This approach is a mechanical one that views joints (whether hinge or ball-and-socket types) as wheels and muscles as a load needing to be stretched on a pulley-like system (see fig. 4.1 on page 72).

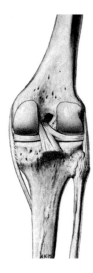

Fig. 4.1. Stretching improves functioning of joints such as the knee.

Laboratories studying muscles have found that they are most efficient at particular lengths. In general, the shorter the muscle's length, the less strength it has. On the other hand, there is a point at which a muscle that is elongated excessively loses strength (fig. 4.2). (This overstretching is unlikely to occur with limb musculature during warm-up activities.) Stretching allows optimum functioning of muscle fibers by placing them at their ideal length.

Muscles around a joint are classically described in terms of the agonists and antagonists for each possible motion. From a Western viewpoint, optimal muscle contraction can only happen when the

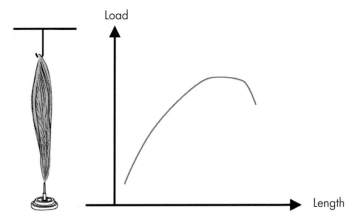

Fig. 4.2. Graph showing ideal muscle length against load

antagonists relax and allow the movement to occur unimpeded. This involves stabilizing the particular joint. From a Western viewpoint, stretching promotes relaxation of the antagonists so that the agonists are not impeded. Stretching also helps the proprioceptors read muscle lengths and degrees of relaxation in order to coordinate the complex movements optimally.

This Newtonian model is initially useful, but it breaks down under careful thought: real-life moves are never performed in such isolated and localized scenarios. Even the most simple Tai Chi or martial move uses the whole body. Wu Yu-Hsiang says, "Remember when moving, there is no place that does not move."[8] Furthermore, most moves are too complex for the intellect to initiate and coordinate. Imagine having to think all of this to execute a palm strike: "contract rhomboids, relax pectorals, while simultaneously extending the shoulder with the triceps, stabilize the elbow with flexors and extensors while contracting the extensors of the forearm to extend the wrist and then perform the sequence in its reverse." Western models are useful for laboratory analysis but they do not necessarily assist the adept in coordination of movement. We need something simpler yet more profound.

What does a tiger think when it's pouncing on its prey, or a deer when it is fleeing and running? The answer we all know is—not much! For animals, movement is a function of the lower brain. It is the higher functions that have disturbed our innate coordination. Therefore, perhaps the answer lies in the process of undoing and unthinking. It is about returning to nature and simplicity and turning off our intellect. Lao Tsu says:

> *Empty yourself of everything.*
> *Let the mind rest in peace.*
> *Returning to the source is stillness.*
> *Which is the way of nature.*[9]

From an Eastern perspective, the fragmentation of imagination, thought, breath, sensation, and muscular contraction have to be reduced. Stretching accomplishes this by opening chi channels, allowing the movement of chi and jin in the body, and helping us on the journey back to the source. We integrate the mind with the limbs, join imagination to movement, merge the inner senses of the head with the sensations in the limbs, and interweave all of these aspects with the breath. All sensations (or consciousness) are merged into one experience, usually described as chi, jin, or energy.

In order to stretch in an Eastern way, the intellect (monkey mind) and li (muscular) power need to be turned off. One can imagine or visualize the limbs becoming long while allowing the chi and jin to elongate selected muscle groups (fig. 4.3). Jin can get involved as the breath almost ceases and a powerful force rises through the body, expanding the tan tien and creating a strong whole-body stretch.

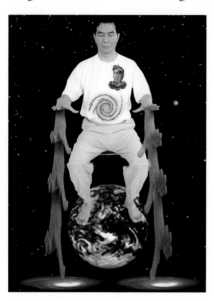

Fig. 4.3. Lengthening a limb with the imagination

Calisthenics and Plyometrics

Calisthenics and plyometrics are used in competitive sports and in external martial arts. They tend to be de-emphasized in internal martial arts as they can interfere with the subtle coordination of spirit, mind, chi, and jin. However, they can play a role for those students who are increasing their aerobic stamina in the Wu style boxing arena.

Rotations

From a Western perspective, rotations are useful for releasing and warming both synovial fluid and the soft tissues. From a Taoist perspective, rotations are used to open the chi meridians within the rotated limb. They can also build up Wei Chi (defensive Chi) around the body. In the Chen school, rotations were used for silk reeling (fig. 4.4). Chen Xin described and drew diagrams of the coiling lines of force that envelop the limbs and torso. These evidently created an ideal interaction between flexor and extensor muscle groups.[10] This warm-up is most beneficial when chi is allowed move the limbs rather than li power.

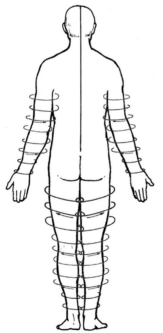

Fig. 4.4. Silk-reeling lines in the body

Percussion

Percussion is a technique taught in the Bone Marrow Nei Kung practice.* It involves percussion with heavy metal wires—although bamboo,

---

*For more information about these percussion practices, see Mantak Chia, *Bone Marrow Nei Kung* (Rochester, Vt.: Destiny Books, 2006).

rattan sticks, or even the hands can be used as well (fig. 4.5). Percussion is seen as a technique to remove stagnant and toxic chi. It also warms up the Iron Shirt function of protecting the body from external blows.

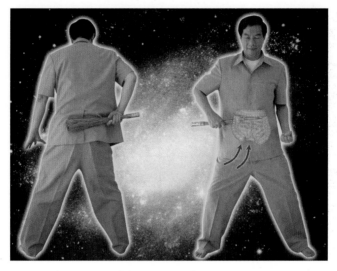

Fig. 4.5. Wire hitting

Shaking and Bouncing

Shaking and bouncing are great ways to warm the tissues of the body and remove stagnant energy from the channels and organs (fig. 4.6). These activities warm the tissues and open channels without the risk of muscle injury associated with stretching and calisthenics. Because bouncing and shaking can damage tissues that are tight or contracted, remember to bounce and shake only in neutral joint positions.

STUDENTS WITH INJURIES

It is rare that someone is in perfect health with no problem areas of pain, stiffness, or limited range of movement. Every human being has persistent chi blockages that require attention. Some have progressed to disease that causes chronic inflammation with arthritis, tendinitis, or osteitis. Some of these conditions are posttraumatic, others are related

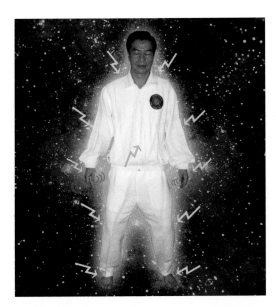

Fig. 4.6. Shaking and bouncing

to innate or acquired inflammatory conditions: all of them deserve respect and nurturing. Inflamed tissues have a low threshold for further damage and inflammation, therefore both the manifestation and the cause of the condition need to be addressed in the warm-up.

With a well-designed warm-up, the cause or root of a condition can eventually heal. For example, tight psoas and piriformis muscles may cause tight adductors of the hip, which in turn result in medial knee pain. While the knee itself does need to be appropriately warmed up, the root of the problem—the tight psoas—also needs to be addressed. Warming up and stretching of the psoas can be accomplished with exercises such as Lifting the Mountain and Monkey Clasps the Knees. The iliopsoas can also be massaged directly using the Empty Force breath in conjunction with abdominal self-massage (Chi Nei Tsang). A tight piriformis can be stretched and then supported by repetitive leg rotations of the silk-reeling type.

A thorough compendium of warm-ups and stretches for the many maladies the body can suffer is beyond the scope of this text. However, we hope that the reader can appreciate the importance of a focused warm-up that caters to the individual and his or her particular conditions.

GENERAL ADVICE FOR WARM-UP ROUTINES

Warm-up routines vary considerably from teacher to teacher and across the various styles. They will also vary according to the physical condition and capabilities of the student. Some students may be at the start of their Tai Chi journey and operate at a purely mechanical and anatomical level, while others will be working to incorporate the higher-level concepts of mind, chi, and jin. Below is a suggested routine that encourages a student to work with spirit and the integrated mind, as well as with chi and jin.

While every warm-up routine will be different, there are some general rules to keep in mind.

Micromovements Are Better than Gross Movements

Very small movements that include internal visualization activate the chi better than ordinary gross movements. Slow is better than rushed. Fast movements in the early stages involve li power and so should be discouraged.

Initiate Movement by Activating the Channels in the Fingers and Toes

To let the chi move you, begin by making subtle movements of fingers and parts of the hand. Distal meridian points (the Jing Well points) activate the chi within each channel.

Rely on the Connection

Focus on staying connected to the heavenly, cosmic, or earth forces rather than on prying open any blockages. Do not try to force open a tense area, just maintain your connections to the energies within and around you. Reinforcing the connections between the limbs is also a useful exercise. Wang Pei-Sheng suggested that his students imagine altering the distance between the shoulder and the hip (Gall Bladder 21 and Gall Bladder 30), elbow and the knee (Large Intestine 11 and Gall Bladder 34), and the palm and the foot (Pericardium 8 and Kidney 1).[11] In closing moves, these points come closer together, while in opening moves they come apart (fig. 4.7).

Larger Joints Lead the Smaller Joints

Large joints lead the medium joints, which in turn lead the small joints. Even though the movement may be initiated by an adjustment

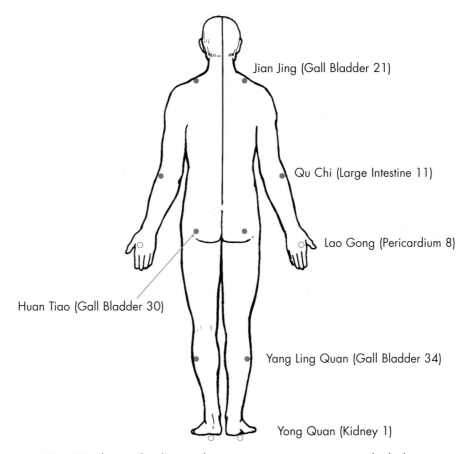

Jian Jing (Gall Bladder 21)

Qu Chi (Large Intestine 11)

Lao Gong (Pericardium 8)

Huan Tiao (Gall Bladder 30)

Yang Ling Quan (Gall Bladder 34)

Yong Quan (Kidney 1)

Fig. 4.7. Altering the distance between acupuncture points on the limbs

of the fingers, the large joints are the first to move according to the laws of chi movement. For example, in raising the arms (like in the opening form of Tai Chi), the chi first opens the armpits, which then raises the elbows, and finally lifts the wrists and hands (fig. 4.8). This is contrary to monkey-mind activity, which usually leads the opposite way—with the small joints.

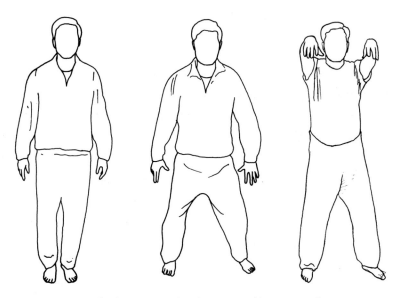

Fig. 4.8. The large joints lead in moves like raising the arms in the opening movements.

Stillness

Stillness is the constancy that connects all the Tai Chi moves and gives rise to the substantial and the insubstantial. Between each routine return to stillness and fill the body with Primordial Chi.

Pleasure

Pleasure is another one of the foundation principles of practice—in warm-ups and in the forms. If a movement feels good, then it is usually right for the body. If something hurts a little, decide if this feels like a nice pain or an awful pain. If it is a nice pain, continue; if it is an awful pain, stop. It is a fine line between pleasure and pain! It is also a fine line between rest and activity. Rest too much and there will be no progress, but if you overtax yourself there will be negative consequences. Remember: it is your body, and ultimately you make the decisions as to the timing and grading of the warm-ups you perform.

Integrate Universal Healing Tao Practices

It is up to the practitioner to integrate practices learned in the Universal Healing Tao system—and outside of it. Initially, the many practices and warm-ups are performed separately, but they can be combined after some time. For example, during stretches, the student can do the Inner Smile meditation and radiate this energy to the desired muscle groups to achieve optimum muscle length and chi flow. The Six Healing Sounds can be practiced if negative emotions arise—though the traditional form and sequence will likely be altered. Sexual practices such as Testicular and Ovarian Breathing or the Big Draw can be practiced in any standing posture. Fusion practices and the Sealing of the Senses can help to improve the student's perception of chi.

Finally, feel free to throw in practices learned from teachers outside the system. Such transplantation and integration of one Universal Healing Tao practice into another is a feature of progress. After a while all the practices melt into one. Yet there will be times when they will need to be practiced in isolation, especially in a group practice.

Play, Be Flexible, and Act According to Whim

Be spontaneous—but only in your home practice! When you are in the presence of teacher, it is time to receive a transmission of chi rather than to explore your personal goals. Group practice relies on group psyche—and group synchronicity—to carry you to new places. It would be disruptive and disrespectful to the teacher and your colleagues to embark on your own tangent. If you do not want to receive the benefits of the class then do not attend!

SUGGESTED WARM-UP ROUTINE TO CULTIVATE CHI AND JIN

The following routine includes a mix of general warm-up exercises along with special attention paid to the cultivation of chi and jin.

 ## Inner Smile and Wu Gong-Tsao's Toy Tumbler

1. Stand with your legs together and palms over the navel. Smile down and fill the organs and the body with heavenly and cosmic chi. Allow the organs to hang freely (fa song).
2. Connect with the earth and root. Allow the earth chi to rise up the body.
3. Let your body begin to rock and sway. Be moved by these forces in a random yet delicate manner. You may simply rock forward and back and side to side, or you may find yourself spiraling like a toy tumbler—spinning more at the head than at the feet (fig. 4.9).
4. As your body becomes loose and free, release your arms and hands and involve them in this exercise.

This Toy Tumbler exercise is a good prelude to the skills used in Iron Shirt training. Form a low center of gravity and find the essence of the heaven, earth, and cosmic forces condensing in the lower tan tien.

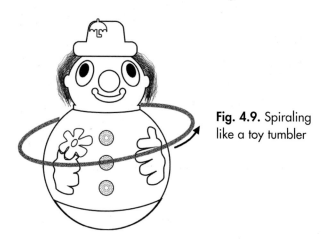

Fig. 4.9. Spiraling like a toy tumbler

Neck

In these simple stretch and rotation exercises for the neck, the aim is not only to stretch the paravertebral and front strap muscles but also to allow chi to open up the space between each vertebra and the base of the skull. This practice has overlap with the Fusion meditations and the spinal cutting exercises.

1. Perform the Crane and Turtle Neck patterns* without involving the thoracic and lumbar spine (fig. 4.10). This is best done extremely slowly. Use the mind to visualize and stretch each small space between the cervical vertebrae.
2. Finish off with rotations clockwise and counterclockwise working up from C7 to C1.

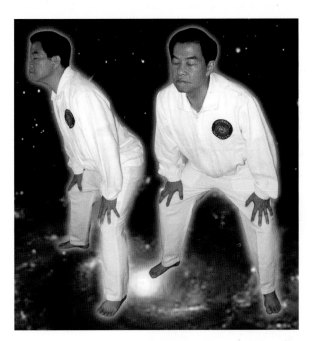

Fig. 4.10. Crane Neck and Turtle Neck patterns

---

*These exercises can be found in Mantak Chia, *Chi Self-Massage* (Rochester, Vt.: Destiny Books, 2006), 57–58.

Spinal Rolldown

The spinal rolldown creates space between all the vertebrae of the spine, similar to what was done with the cervical spine above (fig. 4.11).

1. Start at C1 and slowly roll each vertebra down, bending forward as you go.
2. As you roll down the upper thoracic vertebrae, let the arms hang loose (or lightly clasp your hands) and feel the scapulae relax and fall laterally.
3. Use all your powers of mind to create the song (fa song). Be calm and slow, and have precise internal visualizations as you turn the senses inward.
4. Allow each and every vertebra to flex. You can slightly pack the lower vertebrae to prevent hanging from the hips.
5. Pack the legs by pulling the kneecaps up and externally rotating the hips. In this way, the exercise is full but empty in accordance with the principles of fa song.
6. To end, bend the knees slightly and extend each vertebra back until you are standing vertically again.

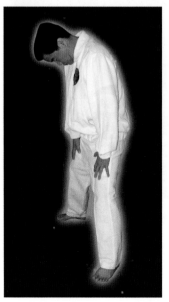

Fig. 4.11. Spinal Rolldown

Arm Rotations and Backbend

In this exercise, use chi and the connection between your palms and the external forces to drive the movement.

1. Stand with legs shoulder width apart with arms at sides and fingers pointed toward the earth. Begin with your palms facing back and allow the chi to move the palms forward.
2. Reach forward and rotate the palms forward, allowing the arms to extend backward.
3. Allow these rotations to get bigger and bigger and higher and higher. Let any stiffness or blocked channels in the shoulder girdle simply melt, by allowing chi to move the palms. Always focus the mind on the connection between the palms and the universe.
4. To end, let your whole body arch backward with the return movement and slightly flex with the forward movement.

 ## Side Torso Stretches

1. Let your fingers open the channels and move the chi, then begin to stretch your torso to the side (fig. 4.12). Make small adjustments of the fingers and palms to initiate significant releases throughout the body. These releases often include the armpits and areas around the pelvis.

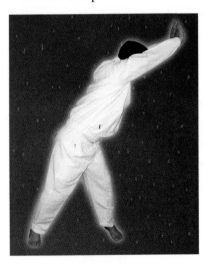

Fig. 4.12. Side stretch with leading palm

2. To extend the stretch further, march the mind down the spinal column, searching for any tense holding patterns. Let the breath be smooth, natural, and calm.

Waist and Pelvis Rotations

Connect to the spiraling energy that rotates the body and Belt channels. Involve the pelvis in these rotations and feel the opening of the lower tan tien, the Belt Channel (Du Mai), and the back and front kuas (fig. 4.13).

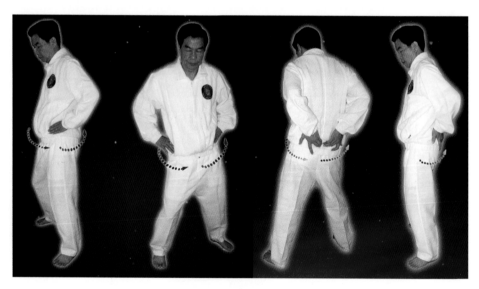

Fig. 4.13. Pelvic rotations

Leg Rotations/Silk Reeling

1. Begin by finding a pleasant sensation—like silk around the foot. This is likely to be some kidney chi.
2. Rotate the foot around and around until more and more of the foot and ankle have this sensation.
3. Wind this sensation upward until it includes the bones and muscles of the lower leg (fig. 4.14).
4. Work harder by moving your hip so that the sensation of silk

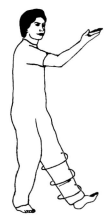

Fig. 4.14. Reeling silk
up the leg

involves the whole of the thigh. This exercise eventually works problem muscles like the psoas and piriformis.

5. Finish off by allowing the chi to move the whole lower limb.

Allowing chi to move the lower limb obeys the same principles as chi moving the upper limb, but it is complicated by the need of the legs to support the body. Work out what adjustments of the feet are necessary for the chi to mobilize the various forms such as the Golden Cock Stands on One Leg, Lotus Kicks, Side Kicks, and so on. These silk reeling warm-up exercises can also be used for the upper limbs as well.

Pelvis and Kua

The adductors, external rotators, and internal rotators of the hip can be stretched with squats, and with postures like Snake Creeps Down, Low Horse stance, and the Golden Turtle. Be mindful of your age, but aim to progress slowly forward. Use the principles of fa song to sink deeper into your stance, and trust that if you go slowly and work with the chi, then you will not suffer an injury.

When working to open the kua, it is helpful to pay attention to your palms: as the palms perform a closing movement, feel the kua open. As the palms open, relax them even more to allow jin to ascend through the structure. It is also helpful to keep in mind the connections between the acupuncture points of the upper limbs and lower limbs as described above on page 79.

A good exercise is to rise and fall in a wide Horse stance, letting your arms rise and fall as well (fig. 4.15). The total movement is similar to a ballet dancer's plié, except that the legs are kept wide apart instead of having the heels together.

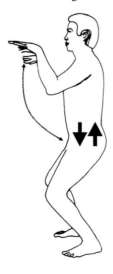

Fig. 4.15. Rising and falling Horse stance with connecting hands

TECHNICAL EXERCISES

Technical exercises are key features of both the Universal Healing Tao system and the Southern Wu style. Technicals can be divided into yin and yang forms, though they are less common in the Yang style.* The yin technicals include variations of Iron Shirt postures and Chi Kung exercises. Yin technicals cultivate the opening of the acupuncture meridians and the strengthening of all aspects of the tan tiens. They improve strength and promote nourishment and the health of the organs. The strength of the tan tien is reflected by the efficiency of the Iron Shirt—which can be tested by the ability to receive body blows or resist pushing. There is considerable overlap between the technical forms of

---

*Although several technicals were mentioned in the *Tai Chi Fa Jin*, many of these are not original Yang style technicals but were included because of the paucity of technicals known in the Yang tradition.

the Universal Healing Tao (UHT) system and the Southern Wu (SW) system. The second column of the table below describes whether the form is an established practice within the Universal Healing Tao system—as part of Iron Shirt or Tan Tien Chi Kung—or alternatively is from the Southern Wu system. The Southern Wu Tang technicals are more oriented to boxing.

TECHNICALS FROM UNIVERSAL HEALING TAO AND SOUTHERN WU STYLE PRACTICES

EXERCISE	UNIVERSAL HEALING TAO OR SOUTHERN WU PRACTICE	TYPE	ASPECT TRAINED
Embracing the Tree	UHT and SW	Yin	Microcosmic Orbit
Holding Golden Urn—Yang	UHT and SW	Yin	Microcosmic Orbit/ Lung and Spleen meridians
Holding Golden Urn—Yin	UHT and SW	Yin	Microcosmic Orbit/ Bladder and Small Intestine meridians
Golden Turtle	UHT and SW	Yin	Open kua and lower tan tien
Buffalo	UHT and SW	Yin	Open kua and front aspect of lower tan tien
Golden Phoenix	UHT	Yin	Packing the three warmers
Iron Bridge (Standing)	UHT and SW	Yin	Conception Vessel
Iron Bridge (Resting)	UHT and SW	Yin	Governing Vessel and Bladder Meridian
Rabbit	UHT and SW	Yin	Front tan tien and Central Thrusting Channel; Xu Jin
Crane	UHT	Yin	Side tan tien and Lateral Thrusting Channels
Bear	UHT	Yin	Back tan tien and Bladder meridian

EXERCISE	UNIVERSAL HEALING TAO OR SOUTHERN WU PRACTICE	TYPE	ASPECT TRAINED
Swallow	UHT	Yang	Sides of the tan tien
Dragon	UHT and SW	Yin	Waist rotation and fist strike; Xu Jin
Eagle	UHT	Yang	Coupling in lower tan tien
Monkey	UHT and SW	Yang	Fa Jin: lower strike; upper and lower tan tien
Elephant	UHT and SW	Yang	Fa Jin: lower strike
Rhinoceros	UHT and SW	Yin	Kua, Small Intestine and Gall Bladder meridians
Horse	UHT	Yang	Fa Jin: close contact (1-inch strike)
Bull	UHT and SW	Yin	Xu and Fa Jin (except phase 8)
Rising and Falling Horse stance	UHT	Yin	Lower tan tien, kua, and Xu Jin
Turning the Wheel	UHT	Yin	Microcosmic Orbit and Xu Jin
Civet Cat	SW	Yang	Fa Jin: fist strike (3-inch punch)
Chopping Wood	SW	Yang	Sinking and downward strikes
Striking to Side	SW	Yang	Sinking and backward strikes
Leading the Goat	SW	Yang	Waist, Central Thrusting Channel, inner wrist
Flicking Fingers	SW	Yang	Fa Jin: fingertips
Swallow Flies through The Clouds (Southern Wu)	UHT and SW	Yang	Fa Jin: side palm strike

Moving Yin Technicals including Silk Reeling

Moving silk reeling technicals are classified as a yin training exercise for the release of discharge power. They are yin because they are done in slow motion. Furthermore, they cultivate softness, fullness, and absorption. They include such forms as the Bull, Jade Rabbit, Turning the Wheel, and Rising and Falling Horse stance. Like general warm-ups, yin technicals also serve the purpose of opening the acupuncture meridians and the three tan tiens.

We hope that the reader understands that yin does not mean weak; by cultivating yin, the practitioner can ensure that the release or yang phase will become more powerful. Silk reeling (chan su jin)[12] is openly taught in the Chen tradition, but moving yin technicals are certainly not unique to the Chen style. Such exercises have been an important aspect of Tai Chi Chuan training in the Yang, Wu, Li, and Sun styles. For example, Li Yi-Yu tells us to "move the chi like coiling silk."[13]

Yin technicals are an alternative to prolonged sitting or standing in Iron Shirt postures; they help open the Microcosmic Orbit, the twelve main acupuncture channels, and the tan tiens. During the yin stages of practice, the body and mind are in an absorptive state that collects chi from the heavens (the sun, moon, planets, and stars) and the earth (five elements of the earthly plane). The three tan tiens are activated to store the jin and chi that are absorbed. Stagnation and blockages are cleared with the gentle movement of chi and jin through the afore-mentioned channels.

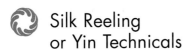 ## Silk Reeling or Yin Technicals

Here are three examples of the slow moving yin technicals. Others can be found in other Universal Healing Tao texts.

❂ Turning the Wheel

The emphasis of this technical is twofold. One is to open all the points of the Microcosmic Orbit (fig. 4.16). The second is to cultivate the appropriate coordination of the whole body—from the feet to the fingertips—in simple circular movements. Jin is released via the vertebral column. The hands are moved by the chi. The novice begins by learning to turn from the waist and release power via the spine. Later, chi is allowed to move parts and then all of the entire structure. Any monkey-mind intention is gradually removed. The following photographs show the external moves, while the diagram shows the movement of focus (the chi ball) within the Microcosmic Orbit.

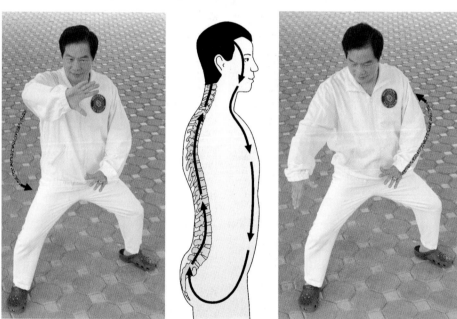

Fig. 4.16. Chi ball within the Microcosmic Orbit

❂ Rowing the Sampan Oars (Bull)

This yin technical includes arm splitting, which is like the breast and butterfly strokes in swimming. The breast stroke variation is better known as Rowing the Sampan Oars. In this particular technical, the

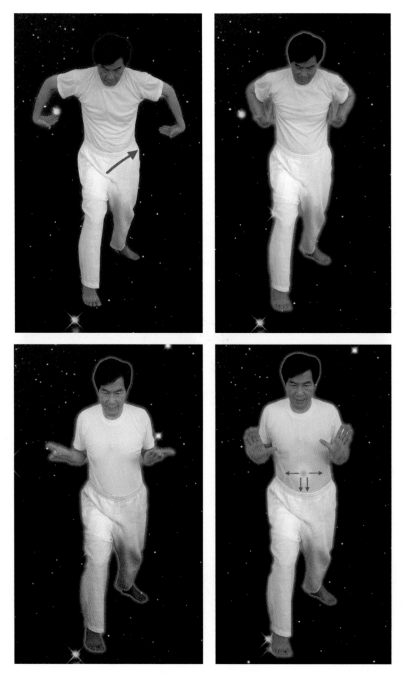

Fig. 4.17. Chi balls with Sampan Oars

tan tien is already forward during the backward movement and hence doesn't require a rotation prior to the discharge of jin. In the butterfly action, however, the focus returns to the standard pattern.

❂ Jade Rabbit Pounds the Drug of Immortality

This technical is done in double-weighted Horse stance only. It works on opening the Central Thrusting Channel (Chong Mai). Again, the principle of allowing the chi to move the limbs is important.

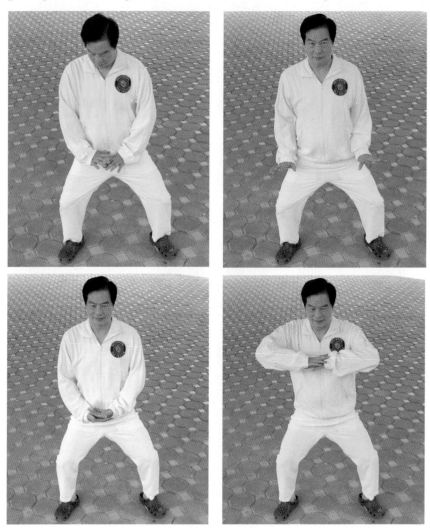

Fig. 4.18. Jade Rabbit opens the Central Thrusting Channel.

Yang Technicals

Yang technicals are more focused on cultivating the power necessary for strikes and blocks within the boxing repertoire. They help the adept relax and use the torque that is created in the waist and lower tan tien. Most spin around the Central Thrusting Channel, gradually dispelling excessive tension that impedes the power of the strike. These exercises include the Swallow, Chopping Wood, the Elephant, Leading the Goat, Backward Striking, Civet Cat Catches the Rat, and Flicking Fingers.* Here are some examples of the yang technicals.

Discharge Power Yang Technicals

These technicals are carried out in fast martial speed.

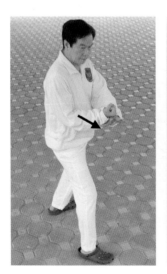 Civet Cat Catches the Rat

Civet Cat Catches the Rat cultivates the Peng force and works all phases of the Fa Jin sequence. This is the classic exercise for development of the "three-inch punch." Power is released from a standing start. The opposition of the force comes from the other arm and its sudden release can create a strong springlike release that is almost impossible to defend. Visualize and imitate nature by capturing a "rat" as you move your fist from an open palm to a closed fist.

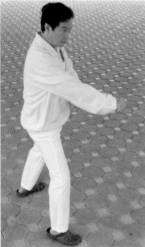

Fig. 4.19. Civet Cat Catches the Rat

---

*See *Tan Tien Chi Kung* and *Tai Chi Fa Jin*. Other yang technicals can be found in *Tan Tien Chi Kung*.

⚙ Chopping Wood

Chopping Wood cultivates Fa Jin in a downward direction. The force is released downward with 90 percent of the weight on one leg. There is a simultaneous sinking of the weight with each strike. The sinking of the weight implies that the weight of the practitioner is transferred with the strike. So not only is there the power generated from the tan tien and arms but also from the body weight. Together this creates a powerful destructive strike. This force is useful in executing the Tsoi force. The name of this technical encourages the same principle as an axe chopping wood: the weight should be more in the hand than in the elbow or shoulder. Maximal power comes from being loose and relaxed.

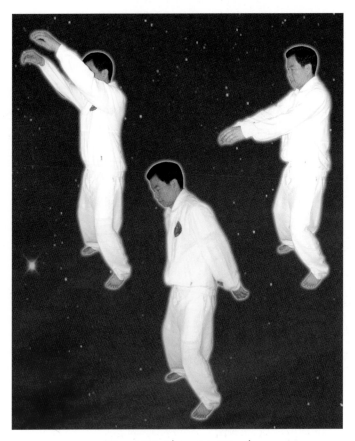

Fig. 4.20. Chopping Wood

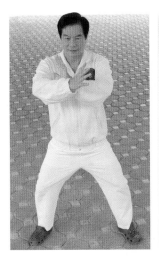
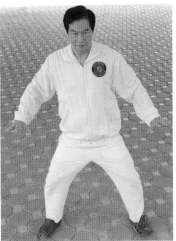

Fig. 4.21.
Striking to Side

⊛ Striking to Side

In this technical, Fa Jin is released simultaneously with two arms to the back. There is the same sense of releasing power via the spine as in the fundamental form of Tai Chi Chi Kung.

⊛ Leading the Goat

Here power is released along the radial side of the forearm. Power is generated as per a Roundhouse Punch or strike. Power is generated through rotation of the Central Thrusting Channel and the movement of focus from the side to the central tan tien. The use of the Yi power is encouraged via the image of "Leading the Goat."

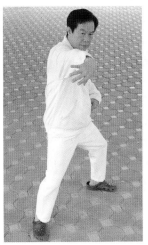
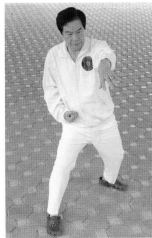

Fig. 4.22. Leading the Goat

❂ Flicking Fingers

This technical really encourages relaxation or fa song while striking. Chi is generated from the tan tien, then reaches the fingertips like a whip. The light yet small fingers are a dangerous weapon as they can be used to strike the eyes or sensitive parts of the face.

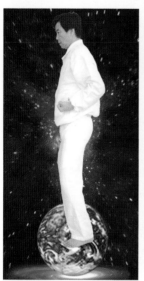 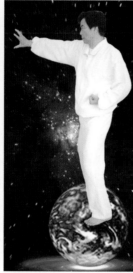

Fig. 4.23. Flicking Fingers

❂ Swallow Flies through the Clouds

This technical works on striking power at shoulder height to the side. It works rotation around the Central Thrusting Channel while allowing soft yin alternation of the arms to enter the upper striking position.

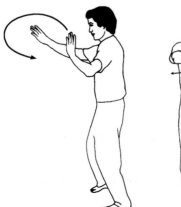 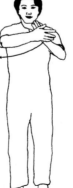

Fig. 4.24. Swallow Flies through the Clouds

Eight Gates with Visualizations

Wu Gong-Tsao discusses these gates in "The Secrets of Eight Techniques" chapter in his "Lecture on Taijiquan,"[14] where he suggests visualizations to help develop each gate. These gates match the teachings within the Yang school as documented by Tan Meng-Hsien.[15]

The Eight Gates with Visualizations

Gate 1: Peng

Begin on the right side. Practice Peng with a movement like a floating boat supported by the water beneath. When the tan tien feels like it is naturally exploding, visualize it as a loaded spring releasing (fig. 4.25). The aim is to follow the release in a relaxed manner.

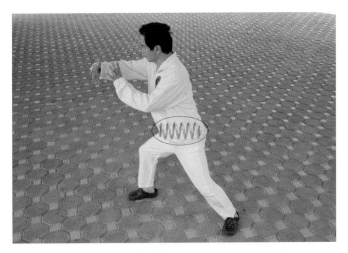

Fig. 4.25. Core spring in the tan tien

Gate 2: Lu

Roll back and sink deeper into your structure as per the Push Hands routine, keeping the kidneys full and the spine straight. Become empty and visualize yourself floating in deep outer space (see fig. 4.26 on page 100). In many respects, Lu represents the first half of the Fa Jin sequence. It can be used on its own to topple an opponent who expects resistance and consequently uproots himself when none is offered.

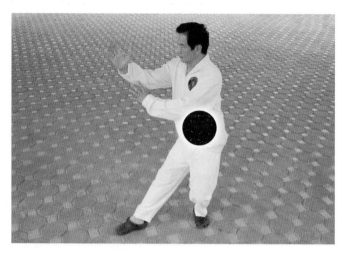

Fig. 4.26. Tan tien as empty outer space

Gate 3: Ji

In this exercise, imagine that the tan tien or the body is connected to two different forces, symbolized by the left and right arms. These two forces then create a reaction at the zenith of the movement that is like bouncing a coin off a hollow and tight drum (fig. 4.27).

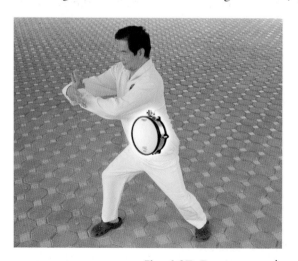
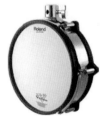

Fig. 4.27. Tan tien as a drum

✷ Gate 4: An

In the yang phase, visualize the energy like water in an outgoing tide—a steady force that fills every defect in the opponent's structure without effort (fig. 4.28). At the moment when the tide seems full—when there can be no more resistance and the opponent is on the verge of imbalance—then release a final surge of jin.

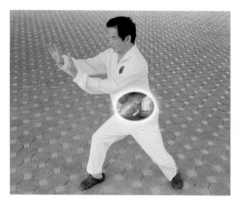

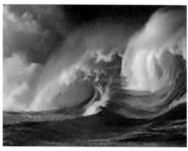

Fig. 4.28. Tan tien as a wave in the sea

✷ Gate 5: Tsai

Visualize yourself and your opponent in a lever position with a defined fulcrum (fig. 4.29). The wrist, elbow, and shoulder can be targets for pressure applied to engage a lock (chin na); finish with discharge power to dislocate a joint or fracture a bone. In this situation, the yin phase breaks the opponent's structure by elongation. In the yang phase (stages 5 to 7), the opponent is set up for the lever. Set up a lever like a balance scale so that only "four ounces" are required to break a "thousand pounds."[16]

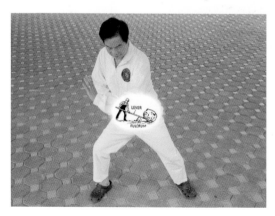

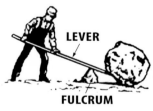

Fig. 4.29. Tsai using the principle of the lever

🌀 Gate 6: Lieh

Next imagine the tan tien like a spiraling vortex or "spinning like a flywheel."[17] The fastest moving point is distant from the central eye of the vortex (fig. 4.30). Any force that entangles itself on the outside of this vortex is cast off a thousand times faster than it entered.

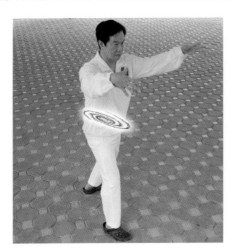

Fig. 4.30. Vortex spiraling in the lower tan tien

🌀 Gate 7: Chou

Visualize the elbow's power as coming from the five elements and being absorbed from the six directions (fig. 4.31). This elemental energy reduces to a unity that ultimately explodes via the elbow joint.

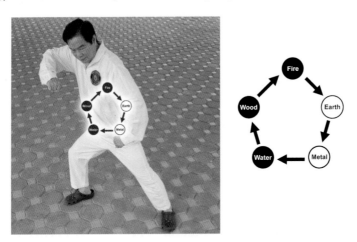

Fig. 4.31. Tan tien absorbing chi from the five elements

☷ Gate 8: Kou

The back and shoulder set up a discharge of power using their weight against an imaginary force—making "a deafening sound like pounding a pestle" (fig. 4.32).[18]

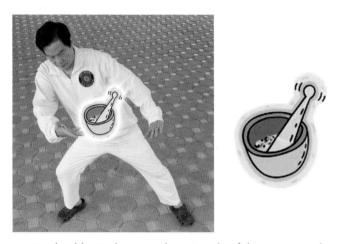

Fig. 4.32. Shoulder Strike using the principle of the mortar and pestle

In these eight gates technical exercises, the eight forces are initially practiced in sequence. (This is opposed to practice or demonstration of the slow form, where the sequence can vary.) In the technical environment, the adept can practice according to his or her own inner timing rather than an imposed time constraint. Multiple repetitions in a relaxed atmosphere allow natural and spontaneous movement of chi and jin to occur. The eight stages of release with four yin and yang stages are initially maintained. However, while building up the chi and jin, the adept may highlight phases 1–4 or 1–7 for a chosen number of repetitions. When the jin has built up and can no longer be contained, it is released.

With further years of practice, the gates also merge and can be reduced to three: upward, downward, and angular discharges. Rather than have awareness of actual anatomical body parts, one can move into the subtle realm of chi, jin, and spirit. An attack becomes discharging a chi/jin ball without much more detail than that.

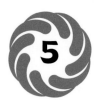

5

The Tai Chi Chi Kung Wu Style Form

This chapter is divided into three sections. The first section describes the Wu Chi stance before the commencement of the form. The second section describes the Short Wu Style Form, which involves the six postures (excluding opening and closing forms) repeated in three directions. The final section is a description of the short form repeated in eight directions.

Beginners and older people generally practice this Tai Chi Chi Kung form with a higher stance. As the student progresses, he or she can practice with a mid-level stance. For martial purposes, one generally uses an extremely low stance.

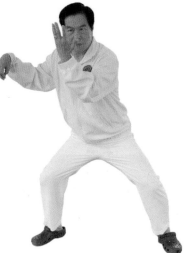

Fig. 5.1. The Tai Chi Chi Kung Wu Style Form

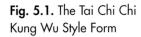

INTRODUCTORY MOVEMENTS

 ## Wu Chi Stance

The first movement of the Tai Chi Chi Kung Wu Style Form is internal, not external. Outwardly, the practitioner stands still, facing north. This position is related to Wu Chi, the primordial unmanifest state (fig. 5.2).

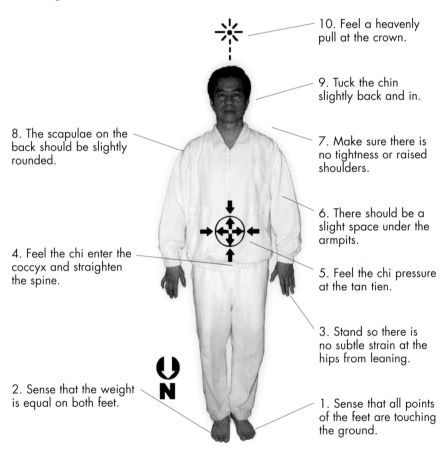

10. Feel a heavenly pull at the crown.

9. Tuck the chin slightly back and in.

8. The scapulae on the back should be slightly rounded.

7. Make sure there is no tightness or raised shoulders.

6. There should be a slight space under the armpits.

4. Feel the chi enter the coccyx and straighten the spine.

5. Feel the chi pressure at the tan tien.

3. Stand so there is no subtle strain at the hips from leaning.

2. Sense that the weight is equal on both feet.

1. Sense that all points of the feet are touching the ground.

Fig. 5.2. Wu Chi Stance

1. Stand with your feet close together, but not touching at the ankles. The nine points of the feet should make contact with the ground. This is the root—the connecting point with the earth energy.

2. Keep your back straight and relaxed and the knees straight, but not locked. No pressure, tension, or pain should be felt in the lumbar area.

3. Relax your shoulders and pull your head upward at the crown. This is the heavenly pull that draws the earth energy up through the feet.

4. Feel the heavenly pull, as if a chi ball above your head is pulling you up. The pull also stretches your spine, allowing the energy to circulate more freely. At the same time, feel the chi enter your coccyx and straighten your spine.

5. Keep your eyes open without strain. The focus is directly ahead, to the horizon.

6. Pull your chin slightly backward. This subtle movement opens the base of the skull so the energy can circulate freely up to the crown and down the front of the body.

7. Lightly place the tip of your tongue against the palate at a point that helps induce salivation (fig. 5.3). Your jaw should be relaxed with the teeth lightly touching. If the jaw is biting down hard, there will be tension on the sides of the head and the throat.

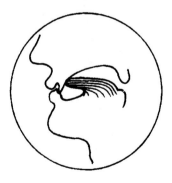

Fig. 5.3. Tongue lightly on the roof of the mouth

8. Relax your throat. Swallow a little saliva and exhale gently to relax the muscles of the neck.

9. The chest should be relaxed and slightly hollowed. This hollowing is produced by a subtle rounding of the scapulae on the back. If the chest is tight, relax it by inhaling gently without making noise and then exhaling just as quietly through parted lips.

10. Breathe deeply and evenly, expanding your abdomen.

11. Bring your attention to your navel or your tan tien. Let the breath penetrate to the tan tien, creating the sensation of a growing energy ball.

12. Relax your arms, leaving a hollow in the armpits as if holding a Ping-Pong ball there. The arms should not be touching the body.

13. Relax the palms of both hands, keeping the fingers loose yet straight. Raise your index fingers very slightly, so you can feel energy sparkling at the tips (fig. 5.4).

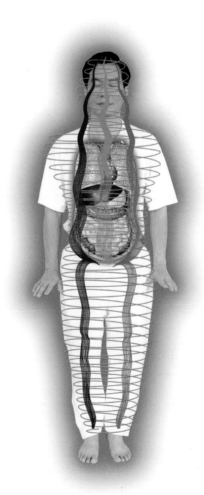

Fig. 5.4. Raise your index fingers to feel the energy spiraling.

14. Feel the palms and soles breathing. Feel the chi ball in the tan tien contracting and expanding with the breath (fig. 5.5).

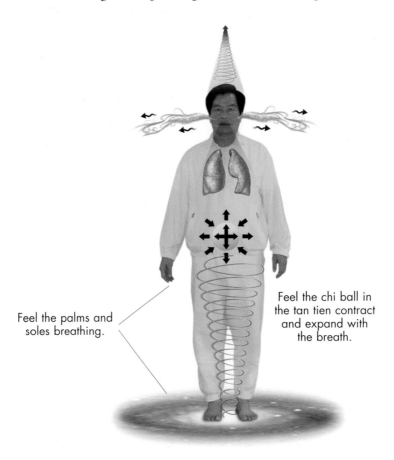

Feel the palms and soles breathing.

Feel the chi ball in the tan tien contract and expand with the breath.

Fig. 5.5. Tan tien breathing

Smile

1. Smile down to the thymus gland below your neck. Allow the smile to spread to your heart and all other organs.
2. Smile down to your navel.
3. Listen to your heartbeat. Follow the pulse from your heart out through the chest, shoulders, upper arms, elbows, forearms, wrists, hands, and fingers. Feel the pulse in the index and pinkie fingers.

Breathing

1. Become aware of the earth energy at your feet, the heavenly pull at your crown, and the cosmic energy in front of your body. Inhale gently without making noise and draw the cosmic energy into the mid-eyebrow point.
2. Let the cosmic energy penetrate deeply into the lungs, then spread to all of your organs. Let it fill the soles of your feet.
3. When your inhalation is complete, retain the breath for a moment without straining, then begin to exhale gently without making noise. Your breath should be so gentle that it would not move a piece of paper placed in front of your nostrils.

THE THREE-DIRECTION SHORT WU FORM

This form begins with step out to the left and an unusual Bend Down form before it proceeds to the core movements.

 Opening the Three-Direction Short Wu Form

🌀 *Preparation: Step Out*

1. As you exhale, begin to sink down, shifting your weight onto your right leg. The sinking should originate from the hips and sacrum, as sinking by simply bending the knees puts too much stress on them, resulting in swelling and injury. Sink and fold at the groin (kua) without much of a bend in the knees, and feel your weight transfer down the back of your knee to the heel (see fig. 5.6 on page 110).
2. Sink your chest and round the scapulae a little bit more, so that your arms come out slightly from your sides. As the chest sinks, the sternum moves inward, massaging the thymus gland.
3. Rotate your hands so that the palms face back. Feel the energy flowing through your arms down to the palms and fingertips.

Opening Movements

4. Begin to shift your weight onto your right leg. Keep your crown aligned with the heavenly force, so there is no leaning to compensate for sinking down on the right leg.

5. When all the weight is on the right leg, inhale as you lift the left heel, keeping the big toe touching the ground.

6. Separate the left leg by brushing the ground lightly with the big toe, as if tracing a line. The separation between the two feet should be roughly the width of the shoulders. This is the base. If the space between the feet is less than shoulder width, the base will be narrower than the top, and the structure will be top-heavy. In this style, the base should not be wider than the shoulders' width.

7. Exhale as you place your left foot at a 45-degree open angle, firmly touching all nine points on the ground. Shift your weight so that it is on both feet equally.

At this point, your knees should remain slightly bent, but not going over the edge of the toes. Your pelvic area is open, and the energy ball

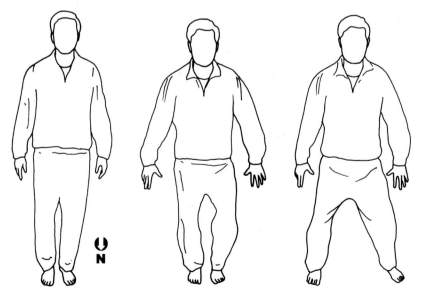

Fig. 5.6. Opening Form

is in the navel area. Your spine should be stretched by the heavenly pull while your sacrum is pulled down by the earth force.

❂ Bend Down

In this move, the practitioner bends face down from the waist, then rises up with the arms forward and finally returns the palms to the side (face down) at the level of the lower tan tien. This move is not present in the majority of Wu forms and is a signature move of the Universal Healing Tao Form.

1. Release the lumbar and lower thoracic vertebrae, and bend 90 degrees forward at the waist, until you are facing the earth with your whole upper torso.
2. Let your hands move straight from your hips to hang down vertically (fig. 5.7).
3. Bend the knees a little more and return to the upright position, keeping your arms forward—with elbows slightly bent—as you straighten up.

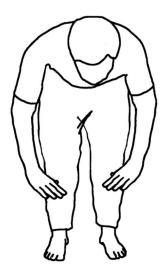

Fig. 5.7. Bend Down

The next sequence is the core part of the Three-Direction Short Wu Form. It starts with a Right-Hand Form facing north, transitions into a Left-Hand Form facing west, and finishes with a Right-Hand Form facing south.

Core Movements: Right-Hand Form, Facing North

The first part of the Three-Direction Short Wu Form is a Right-Hand Form. It begins as you raise your arms back up from the Bend Down position.

☵ *Opening the Right-Hand Form*

1. When your arms reach shoulder height, flex the elbows a little bit to move your palms closer to the shoulders (fig. 5.8).
2. When the arms have reached their peak, lower them—palms facing down—to the level of the navel.

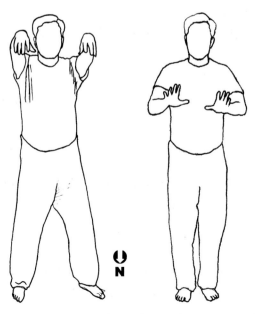

Fig. 5.8. Opening the Right-Hand Form (to north)

Core Movements: Right-Hand Form (Facing North)

⟳ Grasping the Bird's Tail (Right-Hand Form, Facing North)

The spirit of this form is the intention of grasping an elusive and ever-moving bird's tail. The practitioner steps forward with the left leg while the left arm moves forward in a Press position. From there, the waist rotates and the arms parry in the lower and upper positions before ending up in a palm strike. This is different from the Yang form as the spine is slanted, there is no Ward Off, and the form culminates in a single-handed strike rather than a double.

1. Shift your weight to the right leg and step directly forward with the left leg, contacting the earth with your left heel. Rotate the foot to the northeast as the waist moves forward. The arms simultaneously form arcs from the waist, moving sideways, upward, and then inward (see fig. 5.9 on page 114).

2. Lean forward with the spine at an angle and place the toes and soles of your feet on the ground, keeping the left foot facing the northeast. Rest the right palm on the inside of the left wrist to form Press position.

3. Maintaining the feet and weight forward, rotate the waist to the east and make two circles with the arms. During the first circle, parry with the right palm downward, keeping the wrist supported on its radial and palmar aspects by the fingers of the left hand. As the right wrist returns in its circle to the waist, shift your body weight to the back foot while keeping the body structure vertical.

4. During the second circle, make an upward parry with the left fingers supporting the palmar aspect of the right wrist. As the arms move forward, shift your weight again to the front foot. When the arms return, shift weight to the back leg again.

5. Finish the second circular parry with a vertical Palm Strike to the northeast, simultaneously moving your weight to the front (right) leg.

Core Movements: Right-Hand Form (Facing North)

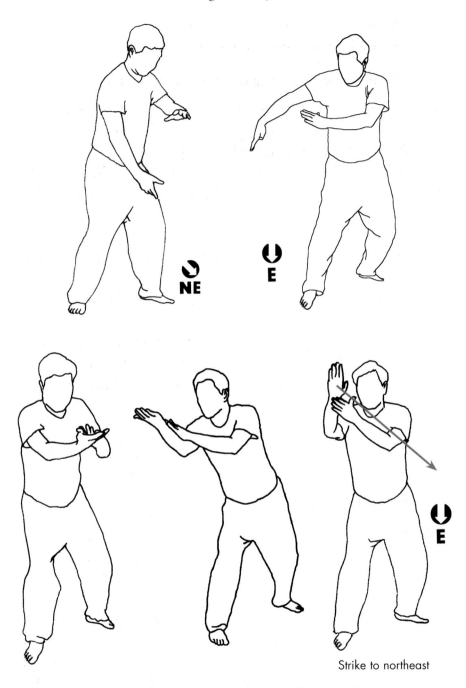

Strike to northeast

Fig. 5.9. Bird's Tail (to east) and Palm Strike (to northeast)

⟳ Single Whip, Flying Oblique, and Lift Hand Step Forward

○ Single Whip (Right-Hand Form, Facing North)

The spirit of this form invokes the Lieh or Splitting Force, which occurs when cracking a whip. In this form, a whip is executed with a hook from the right hand; the left Palm Strike is executed in a double-weighted square Horse stance. This is different from the Yang style Single Whip because it is double-weighted and executed facing midway between the two palms.

1. From the right palm strike in the previous step, rotate the right wrist inward and form a beak (fig. 5.10).
2. Rotate the left foot to the west corner, creating a double-weighted Horse stance.
3. Rotate your waist to move your left palm leftward over your face, then across the front of your body until it is a foot past the left shoulder. Keep the right-hand beak about a foot past the right shoulder.

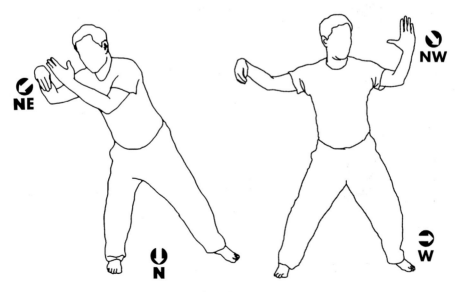

Fig. 5.10. Single Whip (to northwest)

Core Movements: Right-Hand Form (Facing North)

To execute the attacking aspect of this form, rotate the waist back to the right (gaze following), striking to the north with the left vertical open palm.

○ Flying Oblique (Right-Hand Form, Facing North)

This form invokes the spirit of the mythical roc—a bird of prey. The practitioner mimics the bird flying through the sky. In this form, the left attacking arm is held above the head, while the defensive right palm is outside the right thigh. It is different from the Yang form as the body is leaning back with the shoulders behind the buttocks; in the Yang form, both weight and intention are forward.

4. Shift weight slightly onto the left leg, and allow the waist to rotate to the left (fig. 5.11). At the same time, move the right palm leftward across the body, crossing over above the left arm as you open

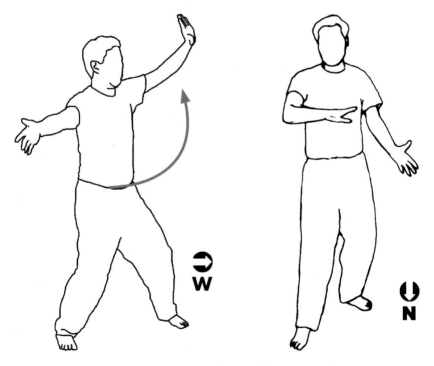

Fig. 5.11. Moving into Flying Oblique (to north)

Core Movements: Right-Hand Form (Facing North)

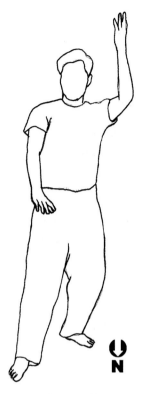

Fig. 5.12. Flying Oblique (to north)

the right palm downward. Straighten the right knee and point the toes somewhat.

5. Rotate the waist and gaze to the right (north) and lean your trunk slightly backward (fig. 5.12). Raise your left arm above your head—palm facing the body—as you bring the right palm down to the outside of the right hip.

○ Lift Hand Step Forward
(Right-Hand Form, Facing North)

The spirit of this form is found in its martial moves: one in which the right palm leads a Press and the other in which an upward wrist (back) or palm performs a strike.

6. From the Flying Oblique position, bend forward and place your weight onto the right (front) bent leg. Move your hands into a Press-like position with the right palm most outward and facing the chest. Direct your gaze to the right palm (fig 5.13).

7. Stand up by bringing the left leg parallel to the right, shoulder width apart. Straighten the right arm as you raise the palm to the sky and follow it with your gaze. At the same time, move the left hand, palm down, to the left side of the hip.

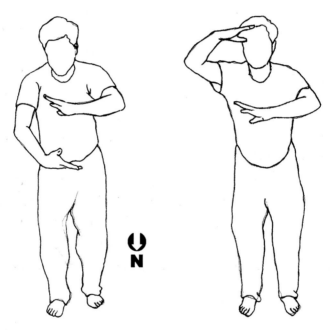

Fig. 5.13. Lift Hand Step Forward (to north)

❂ White Crane Spreads Its Wings (Right-Hand Form, Facing North)

This form invokes the spirit of the white crane—associated with longevity and immortality—stretching and spreading its wings. The whole trunk does a sweeping movement down and to the left while the arms spread open. Finally, the body and arms return to a neutral position preparing for the next form (Brush Knee). It is different from

Core Movements: Right-Hand Form (Facing North)

the Yang style, which spreads the arms in a stretched vertical plane and has no bending of the waist.

1. Bend forward again, moving your hands into the same Press-like position—with the right palm most outward and facing the chest. Keep your gaze just beneath the right palm (fig. 5.14).

2. When your trunk has reached a 90-degree angle from the legs, rotate your waist to the left and simultaneously spread your arms to the sides. The palms should face almost downward, with the left fingertips facing north and the right fingertips facing west. Rotate your gaze to the west—at approximately waist height—toward an imaginary opponent.

3. Straighten up to the opening stance, keeping the legs parallel and shoulder width apart. Rotate the waist northward as you move your arms back alongside the trunk, to a ready position for the Brush Knee strike.

4. Swing your left arm northward, shifting the elbow closer to the ribs as your rotate the palm outward facing north, at heart level. At the same time, rotate the right palm inward to face the chest at shoulder height. Return your gaze to the north, looking over the palms. Keep your weight distributed evenly on both legs.

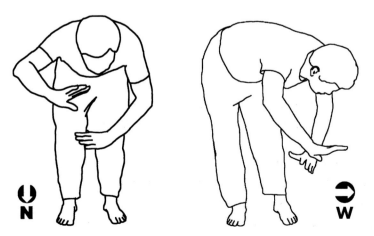

Fig. 5.14. White Crane Spreads Its Wings (to north)

Core Movements: Right-Hand Form (Facing North)

☯ Brush Knee
(Right-Hand Form Facing North)

The spirit of this form is purely a martial one—the right palm attacks the face or chest while the left palm executes a lower block. The form is similar to the Yang style, except that the frame is small and hence the legs are closer together. Because the stance is high, the palm no longer brushes the knee and instead moves across the waist. The spine is also angulated forward in contrast to the Yang vertical position. The palm strike remains angular, with little emphasis on the heel palm strike compared to the Yang style.*

1. Shift all of your weight onto the right leg and lift the left foot off the ground. At the same time, rotate your gaze and your waist to the right as you draw a loop with the right palm, turning it upward and then downward (fig. 5.15).

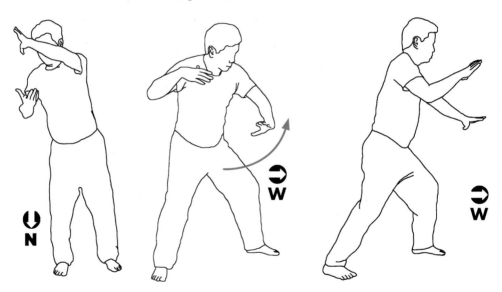

Fig. 5.15. Brush Knee (to west), transitioning to Left-Hand Form to west

*There are differences between the Northern and Southern Wu styles with the Brush Knee. As discussed in chapter 1, the Northern Wu has its signature preparation position as a cocked wrist juxtaposed to the ear. The Southern school remains closer to the Yang style.

Core Movements: Right-Hand Form (Facing North)

2. Rotate your waist and gaze to the west as you place your left heel in the southwest corner, about a shoulder's width from the right heel. Move your right palm horizontally forward at shoulder height until the elbow is only slightly bent. At the same time, draw an arc with the left palm (facing down) from the shoulder to a position outside the left hip.

Core Movements Left-Hand Form, Facing West

In this sequence, the forms are exactly the same except for the following: the sequence begins with Grasping the Bird's Tail, skipping the Opening and Bend Down forms. All moves have interchanged left and right sides. The Single Whip is different, as it now involves stepping out in a 90-degree arc—placing the leading leg in the southeast corner—instead of remaining stationary as it does in the first part. Note that in the Flying Oblique, the right arm—not the left—moves above the head. Furthermore, the leading leg in Brush Knee makes a 180-degree step to the southwest corner.

This section will highlight the Iron Shirt and chi movement principles involved with each form. This will benefit the reader who broadly understands the moves but wants to develop internal power.

🌀 *Grasping the Bird's Tail (Left-Hand Form, Facing West)*

1. Perform a lower parry and an upper parry facing the west (see figs. 5.16 and 5.17 on page 122).
2. Finish the second circular parry with a Palm Strike to the northwest, simultaneously letting your weight shift to the front (left) leg. Let your right hand drift across your body (palm facing down) to join the left wrist. The next form is then commenced.

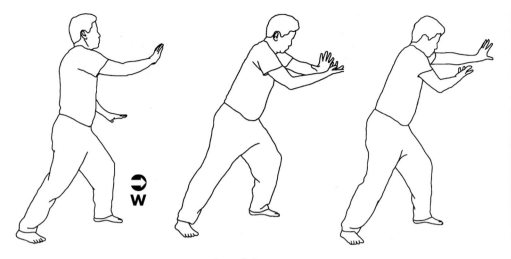

Fig. 5.16. Bird's Tail (lower parry to west)

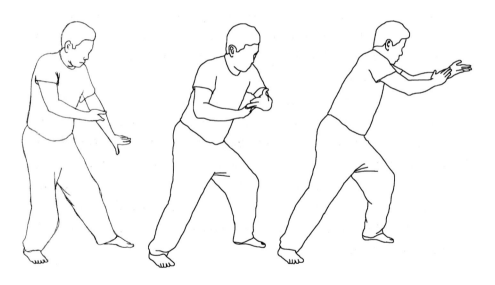

Fig. 5.17. Bird's Tail (upper parry to west)

In this form, the tan tien rotates in a counterclockwise direction with the sensation of rolling a chi ball in the Belt Channel. This is done as the weight is transferred from the front to the back foot.

Core Movements: Left-Hand Form (Facing West)

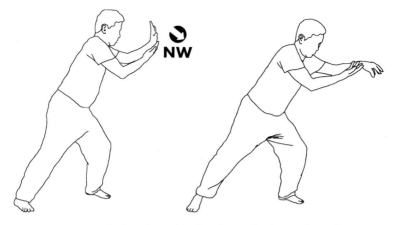

Fig. 5.18. End of Bird's Tail with Palm Strike (to northwest)

When the weight is back, remember that the kidneys should be full. No matter whether the weight is forward or back, all Iron Shirt principles must be maintained. Theoretically, a push by an opponent at any stage would be able to be received and managed. The student should notice that with the upper parry, the chi ball rises to the solar plexus Belt Channel.

The vertical Palm Strike is directed toward the northwest corner rather than toward the left (west) as would be expected if following the same pattern as in the preceding Right-Hand Form (fig. 5.18); the left foot rotates from the west to the northwest as well. The Palm Strike uses all of the discharge principles as jin moves from the earth through the legs—keeping the coccyx tucked in, opening the kua, and passing jin through the spinal column and out through the curved arms.

Single Whip, Flying Oblique, and Lift Hand Step Forward

Single Whip (Left-Hand Form, Facing West)

1. Form a beak with the left hand and direct it to the northwest (see fig. 5.19 on page 124).

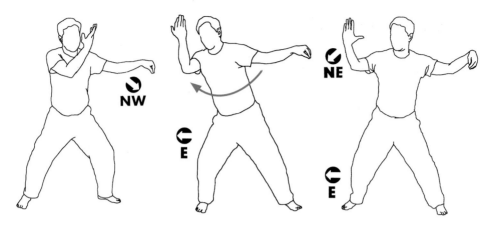

Fig. 5.19. Single Whip (to northeast)

2. Place the right foot pointing almost directly east and complete the Single Whip facing northeast.

In the Single Whip the waist is loaded like a coiled spring around the Central Thrusting Channel, then released without effort. In the slow form, the practitioner should feel the chi initially descending into the earth, then returning and loading the tan tien by tucking in the coccyx and opening the front kua before releasing the whip.

○ Flying Oblique and Lift Hand Step Forward (Left-Hand Form, Facing West)

3. Shift weight slightly onto the right leg, and allow the waist to rotate to the right. At the same time, move the left palm rightward across the body. Straighten the left leg a little bit.
4. Rotate the waist and gaze to the left and lean your trunk slightly backward. Raise your right arm above your head—palm facing the body—as you bring the left palm down to the outside of the left hip (fig. 5.20).

This move displays the eight stages of releasing jin that were discussed in *Tai Chi Fa Jin*. The first four stages comprise the yin phase,

Core Movements: Left-Hand Form (Facing West)

in this case allowing the chi to move the left arm across the body. This allows the structure to relax and in some respects contract—that is, activate the empty force and feel the coccyx tuck, the navel and chest sink, and the kua open. For a moment this tension resides in the earth—and then the waist rotates. From here, the last four stages execute the yang or attacking component of the move: jin ascends and packs the tan tien, spine, and limbs while the right arm ascends and the left hand protects the lower body.

5. Still facing north, bend forward and place your weight onto the left (front) bent leg. Move your hands into a Press-like position with the left palm most outward and facing the chest. Direct your gaze to the left palm.
6. Stand up by bringing the right leg parallel to the left, shoulder width apart. Straighten the left arm as you raise the palm to the sky and follow it with your gaze. At the same time, move the right hand, palm down, to the right side of the hip.

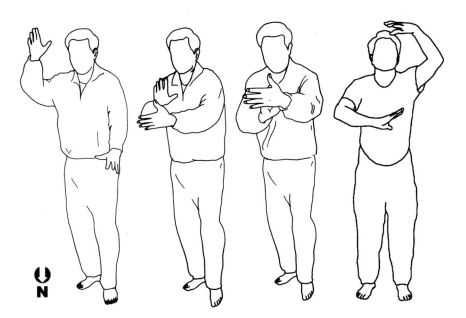

Fig. 5.20. Flying Oblique and Lift Hand Step Forward (to north)

Core Movements: Left-Hand Form (Facing West)

This move demonstrates the principles of the Press, in that excellent timing and structure enable a moment of impact in which the opponent bounces away like a coin hitting a drum. The structure must be absolutely ideal—with legs rooted, tan tien full, and rotation of the waist coinciding perfectly with the placement of the right hand behind the left wrist, while the scapulae remain round and the chin stays tucked in.

◎ White Crane Spreads Its Wings (Left-Hand Form, Facing West)

1. Begin by bending the waist to a 90-degree angle as your arms move down in front of the body, palms facing down (fig. 5.21). Keep your gaze just beneath the left palm.

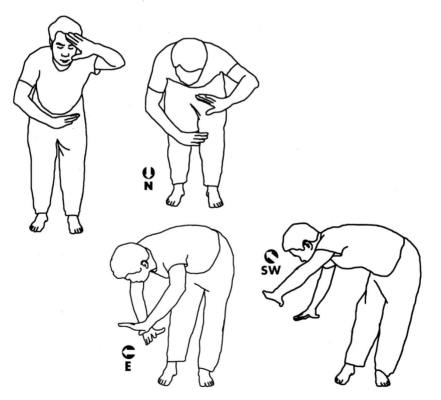

Fig. 5.21. White Crane Spreads Its Wings (to north)

2. When your trunk has reached a 90-degree angle from the legs, rotate your waist to the right (toward the southeast) and simultaneously spread your arms to the sides. The palms should face almost downward, with the right fingertips facing north and the left fingertips facing east. Rotate your gaze to the southeast corner—at approximately waist height—toward an imaginary opponent.

3. Straighten up to the opening stance (fig. 5.22), keeping the legs parallel and shoulder width apart. Rotate the waist northward as you move your arms back alongside the trunk, to a ready position for the Brush Knee strike.

4. Swing your right arm northward, shifting the elbow closer to the ribs as you rotate the palm outward facing north, at heart level. At the same time, rotate the left palm inward to face the chest at shoulder height. Return your gaze to the north, looking over the palms. Keep your weight distributed evenly on both legs.

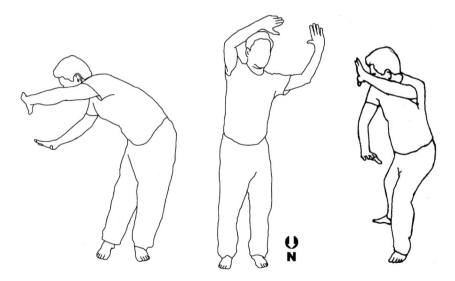

Fig. 5.22. End of White Crane and preparation for Brush Knee

⊙ Brush Knee (Left-Hand Form, Facing West)

The terminal aspect of the White Crane merges into the preparatory or yin phase of Brush Knee. In this form the yin phase includes the forward bend, standing, and the initial rotation of the waist to the right toward the southeast corner (see fig. 5.21), while the attacking power component is the recoil back to the north (shown in fig. 5.22). This will make sense when the martial and spirit aspects are described in the third part. Remember that in the advanced form, the breath is intimately linked to the yin and yang phases of jin and power release (through whole-body breathing). However, beginners may also learn to control the gross breath by inhaling on closing movements and exhaling on outward or attacking movements. Ultimately the breath, mind, jin, and spirit must marry.

1. In order to make this large directional change to the south, pivot your left foot on the heel to the east and place your right heel in the southwest corner about a shoulder's width from the left heel, with your right toes facing south. At the same time, rotate your gaze and your waist initially to the left then rotate to the right as you execute the Brush Knee to the south (fig. 5.23).

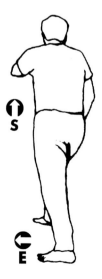

Fig. 5.23. Brush Knee (to south)

2. Move your left palm horizontally forward at shoulder height until the elbow is only slightly bent. At the same time, draw an arc with the right palm (facing down) from the shoulder to a position outside the right hip (fig. 5.24).

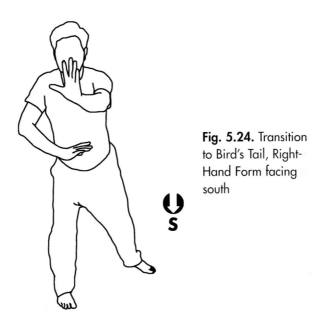

Fig. 5.24. Transition to Bird's Tail, Right-Hand Form facing south

Brush Knee is the classic move for Fa Jin. In the preparation or yin phase, the body relaxes and allows the chi to move the arms and the tan tien. It's as if only an image of the form is held in the mind and it releases the rest of the body. This allows the natural process of power to occur. In this preparation, the empty force allows jin to be stored, then released from the earth in the yang phase—through the legs, spinal column, and arms. In the Wu form—as distinct from the Yang form—the Brush Knee has a descending vector in the Palm Strike as well as the rising jin. This means the body relaxes a little more and sinks at the anticipated moment of impact.

Core Movements:
Right-Hand Form, Facing South

This section will emphasize the spirit and martial aspects of each form while highlighting subtle variations from the two previous cycles.

Grasping the Bird's Tail (Right-Hand Form, Facing South)

1. Move the left palm across and the right hand forward to execute the lower and upper parries (fig. 5.25).

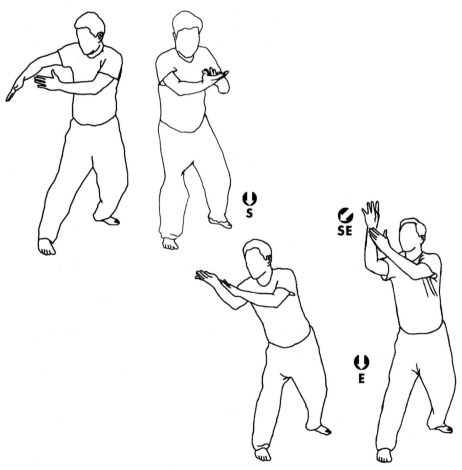

Fig. 5.25. Bird's Tail, Right-Hand Form facing south
(last two figures viewed from east)

2. Finish the second circular parry with a vertical Palm Strike to the southeast, simultaneously moving your weight to the front (right) leg.

The spirit of the Bird's Tail is one of the adept attempting to intercept a flurry of strikes and movements from an imaginary opponent. With this spirit in mind, the gaze and eyes move from lower to upper and to the vertical Palm Strike.

The Bird's Tail with the upper parry is suited to being on the inside of a Roundhouse Punch.* Remember that the Wu boxing style is oriented to close infighting: if you are touching an opponent you can listen and understand through the kinesthetic intelligence of the integrated bodymind. To stand further back and base your actions on visual clues is too slow and awkward for top-level fighting. The spirit of this form should reflect close and tactile intimate fighting.

✪ *Single Whip, Flying Oblique, and Lift Hand Step Forward*

○ Single Whip (Right-Hand Form, Facing South)

1. Make a beak with the right hand in the southeast corner and point the right foot to the east (see fig. 5.26 on page 132).
2. Place the left heel shoulder width apart from the right heel, with the left foot facing north.
3. Rotate your waist to the left to move your left palm over your face, then across the front of your body until it is a foot past the left shoulder. Let your gaze follow the left palm and rest toward the northeast. Keep the right-hand beak about a foot past the right shoulder.

   To execute the attacking aspect of this form, strike to the northeast with the left vertical open palm.

---

*For more information on the boxing applications of the forms, see chapters 7 and 8 in this book.

Core Movements: Right-Hand Form (Facing South)

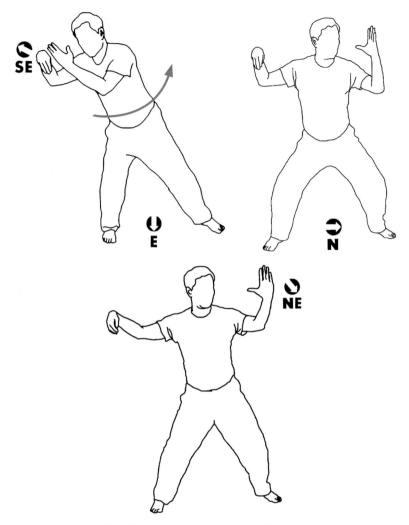

Fig. 5.26. Single Whip (to northeast)

The spirit of this form is to mimic in slow motion the action and sound of a whip. Imagine listening to the sound and feel the action of the whip while executing this move.

From a martial perspective, the stationary side of the whip—the beak and the open palm—becomes the devastating end. The beak grounds the attack as it grapples or connects with the opponent's arm, while the palm strikes the face or torso. Make an effort to visualize and feel the opponent's arms while performing this move.

Core Movements: Right-Hand Form (Facing South)

○ Flying Oblique (Right-Hand Form, Facing South)

4. Shift weight slightly onto the left leg, and allow the waist to rotate to the left (fig. 5.27). At the same time, move the right palm leftward across the body, crossing over above the left arm as you open the right palm downward.

5. Rotate the waist and gaze back to the right (east), with the right foot facing east and the left foot facing northeast, and lean your trunk slightly backward. Raise your left arm above your head— palm facing the body—as you bring the right palm down to the outside of the right hip.

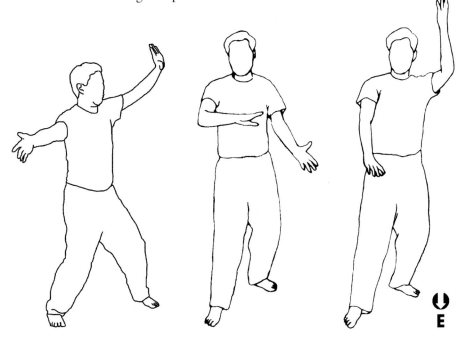

Fig. 5.27. Flying Oblique (to east)

The mind is in a trancelike state at this point, with the subconscious and body senses all activated, and it is possible to channel spirits and deities. This is the time to call upon the power of the roc—a large bird with terrific flying power. Channeling the spirit of the form can improve your form and enhance your power, making you light and agile.

In martial situations, again imagine yourself close to your opponent and use your left shoulder to Kou the opponent off balance.

○ Lift Hand and Step Forward (Right-Hand Form, Facing South)

6. Bend forward and place your weight onto the right (front) bent leg. Move your hands into a Press-like position with the right palm most outward and facing the chest. Direct your gaze to the right palm (fig. 5.28).

7. Stand up by bringing the left leg parallel to the right, shoulder width apart, with both feet facing east. Straighten the right arm as you raise the palm to the sky and follow it with your gaze. At the same time, move the left hand, palm down, to the left side of the hip.

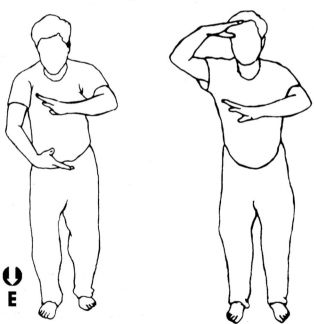

Fig. 5.28. Lift Hand and Step Forward, Right-Hand Form (to east)

This form involves a couple of complex moves facing east, which will be described in more detail in chapter 7 of this book. The first is a Press, wherein the right hand connects with the opponent's left hand. The opponent may attempt to evade by pulling back. Using the principles of Push Hands, the adept can follow this force by executing a Press. If the adept is relaxed, his timing can be perfect: all forces must come together at just the right moment if the opponent is to bounce away like a ball hitting a wall!

Even if this move is unsuccessful, another encounter is possible. As the practitioner stands up, he can strike with the back of the wrist. If still unsuccessful, the palm can turn over and follow the opponent's chin. Despite potential losses, the adept remains calm, maintaining an attitude of eventual accomplishment.

White Crane Spreads Its Wings (Right-Hand Form, Faing South)

1. Bend forward again, moving your hands into the same Press-like position—with the right palm most outward and facing the chest. Keep your gaze just beneath the right palm (see fig. 5.29 on page 136).
2. When your trunk has reached a 90-degree angle from the legs, rotate your waist to the left and simultaneously spread your arms to the sides. The palms should face almost downward, with the left fingertips facing north and the right fingertips facing west. Rotate your gaze to the northwest—at approximately waist height— toward an imaginary opponent.
3. Straighten up to the opening stance, keeping the legs parallel and shoulder width apart. Rotate the waist eastward as you move your arms back alongside the trunk, to a ready position for the Brush Knee strike.

In this form, imagine yourself as a white crane turning and spreading its wings. It should be an effortless movement that has the spirit

Core Movements: Right-Hand Form (Facing South)

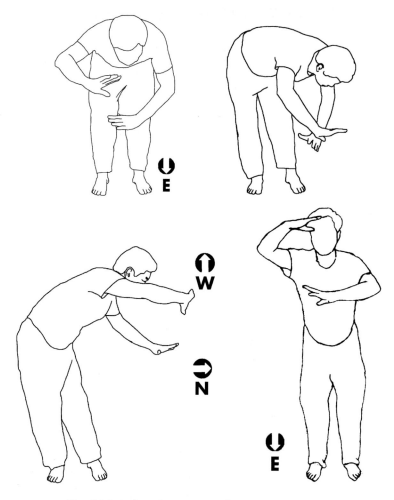

Fig. 5.29. White Crane Spreads Its Wings (to east)

of grace and royalty. The Crane was often used for modeling evasive techniques in martial arts; the bending forward and rotation can be seen as artful dodging culminating in an offensive technique using the Tsai force (lever power) to attack an elbow or shoulder. This move occurs facing the east.

Core Movements: Right-Hand Form (Facing South)

☯ Brush Knee (Right-Hand Form, Facing South)

1. Swing your left arm northward, shifting the elbow closer to the ribs as your rotate the palm outward facing north, at heart level. At the same time, rotate the right palm inward to face the chest at shoulder height. Return your gaze to the north, looking over the palms. Keep your weight distributed evenly on both legs (fig. 5.30).

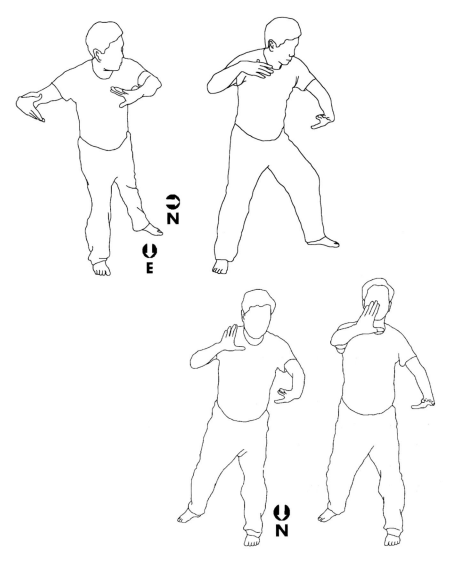

Fig. 5.30. Brush Knee to the north (first two images viewed from east)

2. Shift all of your weight onto the right leg and lift the left foot off the ground. At the same time, rotate your gaze and your waist to the right as you draw a loop with the right palm, turning it upward and then downward.

3. Rotate your waist and gaze to the north as you place your left heel in the north corner, about a shoulder's width from the right heel. Move your right palm horizontally forward at shoulder height until the elbow is only slightly bent. At the same time, draw an arc with the left palm (facing down) from the shoulder to a position outside the left hip.

From parallel feet facing the east the left heel steps to the north and executes a Brush Knee attack. As mentioned above, this form has no spirit link to any animal and merely performs a martial form. Remember that the left palm simultaneously defends while the right palm attacks the face or chest. Please keep this martial spirit alive throughout all forms. Remain alert and release the spirit of the warrior through the eyes and every move.

⊚ Completion: Closing Form

1. Bring the left foot back into alignment with the right leg. The feet should now be parallel and shoulder width apart, facing north (fig. 5.31). At the same time, float your arms out to the sides and then downward, palms facing down. When the palms are alongside the waist at navel height, the leg should finish moving and the feet should be firmly planted.

2. Rotate the palms inward and upward to solar plexus level, so that one palm is under the other facing skyward. At the same time, draw the right foot in close to the left.

3. Straighten your knees to stand up, then bring your arms down— palms downward—alongside the hips. Once at the hips, rotate your palms to face the thighs, with fingers pointing to the earth.

4. Place your palms over your navel and collect energy in the lower

tan tien. You have now completed the journey and return to a space of unity—at one with the Tao.

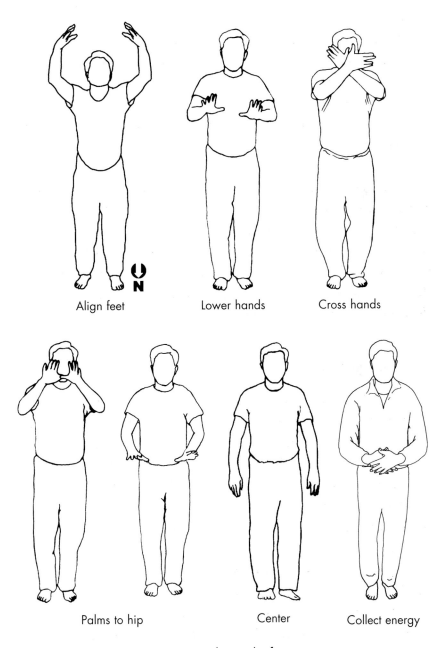

Align feet   Lower hands   Cross hands

Palms to hip   Center   Collect energy

Fig. 5.31. Closing the form

Completion: Closing Form

THE EIGHT-DIRECTION SHORT WU FORM

The Eight-Direction Short Wu Form is a complex form that alternates right- and left-hand sequences. The Right-Hand Forms rotate counterclockwise, while the Left-Hand Forms rotate clockwise. The form ends with closing moves.

 ## Eight-Direction Tai Chi Chi Kung Wu Style Form

Preparation: Step Out

1. Stand facing north with your feet together and knees straight. Feel your head suspended from a string connected to the heavenly force; feel your feet connecting to the earth force.

2. Smile down and inhale. Round the scapulae and sink the chest, and open the armpits. Exhale and sink down, shifting weight onto your right leg. Sink and fold at the groin without much of a bend in the knees, and feel your weight transfer down the back of your knee to the heel.

3. Rotate your hands so that the palms face back. Feel the energy flowing through your arms down to the palms and fingertips.

4. Shift weight to your right leg, keeping your crown aligned with the heavenly force so that you do not lean (fig. 5.32).

5. When all the weight is on the right leg, inhale as you lift the left heel, keeping the big toe touching the ground.

6. Separate the left leg by brushing the ground lightly with the big toe—as if tracing a line—to a point about a shoulder's width apart from the right foot.

7. Exhale as you place your left foot at a 45-degree open angle, firmly touching all nine points on the ground. Shift your weight so that it is on both feet equally.

   At this point, your knees should remain slightly bent, but not

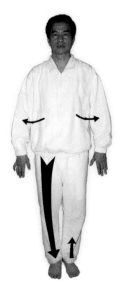

Fig. 5.32. Shifting weight in opening stance in preparation for Step Out

going over the edge of the toes. Your pelvic area is open, and the energy ball is in the navel area. Your spine should be stretched by the heavenly pull while your sacrum is pulled down by the earth force.

8. Bend Down: Lower your upper body from the hips, dropping the head down. (fig. 5.33).

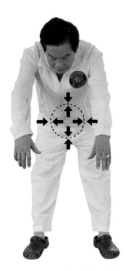

Fig. 5.33. Bend Down

Core Movements

Each corner of the Eight-Direction Form includes a Bird's Tail (which itself includes a Ward Off Strike, a Rollback, and a Press Strike), a Single Whip, a Flying Oblique, Lift Hand Step Forward, and a transition step followed by a Brush Knee.

First Corner, Facing North: Right-Hand Form

This form progresses in a counterclockwise direction.

1. Bird's Tail/Ward Off Strike: Shift your tailbone over the right heel, then draw out and hook your left foot. Form a chi ball with your hands as you Ward Off to the north.

2. Bird's Tail/Rollback: Slide your left fingers to the right wrist and form a circle to the east. At the same time, shift your tailbone over the left heel as you lift up the right heel, opening the hips toward the east.

3. Bird's Tail/Press Strike (to east): Lift your right foot and place the right heel down. Press your left fingers on the right wrist and move forward to the east, then Rollback, sinking back onto the left heel. Pull back the right palm as you push forward to the east, simultaneously shifting your tailbone over the right heel.

4. Single Whip: Form a beak with your right hand as the left foot steps back. Draw your right palm across your face, with eyes following. Strike out to the northwest with palm and beak hands.

5. Flying Oblique: Raise the left palm as the right hand circles downward, crossing at your midsection. Shift tailbone to the right heel.

6. Lift Hand Step Forward: Bend forward with gaze following the right palm. Stand up and bring the left leg forward, shoulder width apart from the right leg. Raise your right hand above your head as the left hand moves to your knee.

7. White Crane Spreads Its Wings: Shift your tailbone to the left heel as you form a chi ball at the midsection with both palms. Draw your right foot up in Iron Shirt stance.

8. Transition: Lower your upper body from the hips, then drop your head as your turn the hips to the left (west). Circle a chi ball over your head to the right side as you shift your tailbone over the right heel.

9. Brush Knee: Step your left heel back toward the south, then turn the right foot 45 degrees to the west. At the same time, drop the left hand so that it brushes the left knee. Shift your tailbone to the center as you push the right hand forward (west).

❂ Second Corner, Facing West: Left-Hand Form

Repeat the sequence above with hands and feet opposite. This form moves in a clockwise direction.

1. Bird's Tail/Ward Off Strike: Shift tailbone to the right heel then draw your left fingers to right wrist and circle forward. Shift the right fingers to the left wrist then circle back.

2. Bird's Tail/Press (to west): Press right fingers forward on right wrist, move hips to west, then circle hips back to northwest for the Palm Strike. Lift left fingers while pushing hips to the west.

3. Single Whip: Form a beak with the left hand as the right foot steps back. Drawing the right palm across with eyes following, then strike out to the northeast with the palm and beak hands.

4. Flying Oblique: Raise your right palm while circling the left hand down, crossing at your midsection. Shift tailbone to left heel.

5. Lift Hand Step Forward: Bend forward with gaze following the left palm. Stand up, bring the right foot forward. Raise your left hand above your head and bring the right hand to your right knee.

6. White Crane Spreads Its Wings: Shift tailbone to left heel as you

form a chi ball at your midsection with both palms. Draw the left foot up in Iron Shirt stance.

7. Transition: Lower your upper body from the hips as you drop your head. Turn hips to the right, circling a chi ball over your head to the left side. Shift your tailbone to the left heel.

8. Brush Knee/Changing Directions (180 degrees): Step back with your right foot pointing to the south. Open hips to south while drawing your right hand down across the waist to protect the right knee. Strike with your left hand to the south.

☯ Third Corner, Facing South: Right-Hand Form

This form moves in a counterclockwise direction.

1. Bird's Tail (to south): Press the left hand south, then shift tailbone to the left heel. Lift your right foot and place the right heel down. Press your left fingers on the right wrist and move forward to the south, then Rollback, sinking back onto the left heel. Pull back the right palm as you push forward to the south, simultaneously shifting your tailbone over the right heel. Move hips 2 counts forward to the south.

2. Single Whip: Form a beak with your right hand in the southeast corner as the left foot steps back. Draw your left palm across with eyes following, then Palm Strike to the northeast with left hand.

3. Flying Oblique (facing east): Raise your left palm, circling the right hand down across the midsection. Shift tailbone to right heel.

4. Lift Hand Step Forward (facing east): Bend forward, with gaze following your right palm. Stand up, bringing the left foot forward. Raise your left hand above your head and move your right hand to your knee.

5. White Crane Spreads Its Wings (facing east): Shift tailbone to left heel, forming a chi ball at the midsection with both palms. Draw the right foot up into Iron Shirt stance.

6. Transition: Lower your upper body from the hips. Drop your

head, then turn hips to the left, circling a chi ball over your head to the right side. Shift tailbone to right heel.

7. Brush Knee (striking north): Step the left heel back to south, then turn the right foot 45 degrees west. Drop the left hand to brush the left knee, then shift tailbone to center and push right hand forward, striking north.

Follow same procedure as south corner (Right-Hand Form) for SE, NW, SW, and NE corners. Begin where the third corner (south) ended.

❂ Fourth Corner, Facing Southeast: Left-Hand Form

1. Bird's Tail to north.
2. Single Whip to southeast.
3. Flying Oblique, Lift Hand Step Forward, and White Crane facing east.
4. Brush Knee strike to southeast, then change direction.

❂ Fifth Corner, Facing Northwest: Right-Hand Form

1. Bird's Tail to southeast.
2. Single Whip to northeast.
3. Flying Oblique, Lift Hand Step Forward, and White Crane facing east.
4. Brush Knee strike to northwest, then change direction.

❂ Sixth Corner, Facing Southwest: Left-Hand Form

1. Bird's Tail to northwest.
2. Single Whip to northeast.
3. Flying Oblique, Lift Hand Step Forward, and White Crane facing north.
4. Brush Knee strike to southwest, then change direction.

⟳ Seventh Corner, Facing Northeast: Right-Hand Form

1. Bird's Tail strike to southwest.
2. Single Whip to southeast.
3. Flying Oblique, Lift Hand Step Forward, and White Crane facing south.
4. Brush Knee strike to northeast, then change direction to north.

⟳ Closing the Form, Facing North

1. Shift tailbone to right hip while releasing the transition. Open both hands, moving them up, outward, and downward.
2. Draw the left foot straight back, setting it down beside the right foot. Shift tailbone to left heel and lift up the right foot, placing it parallel to the left. Draw feet together with toes even.
3. Raise hands 12 inches in front of body to form an **X** below the shoulders (with the left hand closer to your body). Distribute weight evenly between both feet, then simultaneously straighten your body and lower your hands to your sides, with palms facing back.
4. Smile down. Collect energy at the navel.

Eight-Direction Tai Chi Chi Kung Wu Style Form: Angular Directions

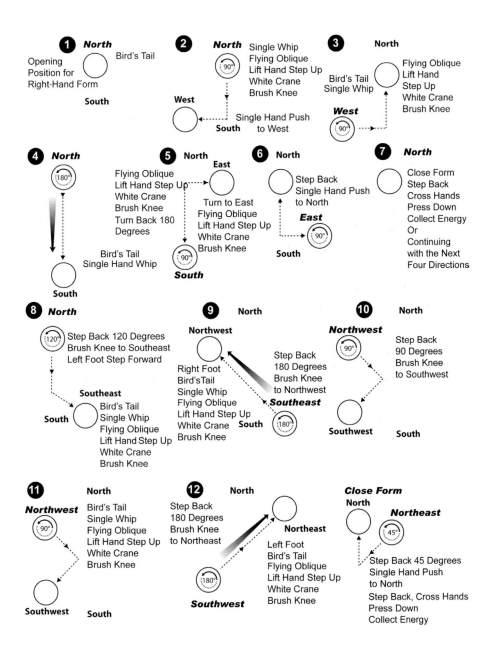

Fig. 5.34. Angular directions for the Eight-Direction Form

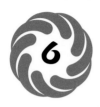

Summary of the Complete Wu Style Form

The following is a simple step-by-step guide to the complete Eight-Direction Tai Chi Chi Kung Wu Style practice. The form will give you the full benefits of Tai Chi Chi Kung.

Opening the Form

1. Beginning Stance: Stand facing north, with your feet relaxed and together. Feel your head suspended from a string connected to the heavenly force.

2. Smile down to your navel, then inhale, round the scapulae, sink the chest, and open the armpits. Exhale and sink down. Shift tailbone to your right heel as you lift the left heel.

3. Inhale and pick up the left foot, then exhale and set down the left foot a shoulder's width apart from the right foot. Stand in Iron Shirt posture.

4. Lower your upper body from the hips and drop your head down.

Raise your upper body and arms from the wrists. Lower your hands.

 ## Core Movements

⟲ *First Round, Facing North: Right-Hand Form*

1. Bird's Tail/Ward Off Strike: Shift tailbone to right heel—draw out and hook left foot forming ball with hands—Ward Off to the north.
2. Bird's Tail/Rollback: Slip left fingers to right wrist forming circle to the east—shift tailbone to left heel and lift up right heel opening the hip to the east.
3. Bird's Tail/Press: Lift right foot and place the right heel down—place left fingers on right wrist and Press forward to the east—Rollback, sinking back on left heel.
4. Bird's Tail/Strike: Pull back the right palm and Push forward to the east, shifting tailbone to right heel.
5. Single Whip: Form beak with right hand to the southeast—step left foot back—draw right palm across with eyes following—strike out to the northwest with palm.
6. Flying Oblique: Raise left palm—circle right hand down, crossing at midsection—shift tailbone to right heel.
7. Lift Hand Step Forward: Raise right hand above head—bring left hand to knee.
8. White Crane Spreads Its Wings: Shift tailbone to left heel forming chi ball at midsection with both palms—draw right foot up—stand in Iron Shirt stance.
9. Transition to Left-Hand Form: Lower upper body from hips—drop head—turn hips to left, circling a chi ball over the head to the right side—shift tailbone to right heel.
10. Brush Knee: Step left heel back to south—turn right foot 45 degrees west—drop left hand, brushing left knee—shift tailbone to center—push right hand forward.

⚙ *Second Round, Facing West: Left-Hand Form*

11. Bird's Tail/Ward Off: Shift tailbone to right heel—draw left fingers to right wrist—circle forward, shifting right fingers to left wrist, then circle back.

12. Bird's Tail/Press: Press right fingers forward on right wrist—move hips to west, then circle hips back to northwest for the Palm Strike.

13. Bird's Tail/Push: Lift back left fingers—push hips to west.

14. Single Whip: Form beak with left hand in northwest corner—step right foot back—draw right palm across with eyes following—strike out to the northeast with palm.

15. Flying Oblique: Raise right palm–circle left hand down, crossing at midsection—shift tailbone to left heel.

16. Lift Hand Step Forward: Raise right hand above head—bring left hand to knee.

17. White Crane: Shift tailbone to right heel, forming chi ball at midsection with both palms—draw left foot up into Iron Shirt stance.

18. Transition to Right-Hand Form: Lower upper body from hips—drop head—turn hips to right, circling chi ball over head to left side—shift tailbone to left heel.

19. Brush Knee/Changing Directions (180 degrees): Step back with right foot pointing south, opening hips to south—draw right hand down (crossing waist) to protect right knee—Press left hand south.

⚙ *Third Round, Facing South: Right-Hand Form*

20. Bird's Tail/Ward Off: Shift tailbone to left heel—circle right hand back across left wrist—shift left fingers to right wrist and circle back.

21. Bird's Tail/Press: With left fingers Press right wrist forward—sink back—shift tailbone to left heel—right hand back.

22. Bird's Tail/Push: Move hips 2 counts forward—to the south.

23. Single Whip: Form beak with right hand in the southeast corner—

step left foot back, drawing left palm across with eyes following—strike out with palm to the northeast.

24. Flying Oblique to east: Raise left palm—circle down right hand crossing at midsection—shift tailbone to right heel.

25. Lift Hand Step Forward: Raise left hand above head—bring right hand to knee.

26. White Crane Spreads Its Wings: Shift tailbone to left heel while forming chi ball at midsection with both palms—draw right foot up into Iron Shirt stance.

27. Transition to Left-Hand Form: Lower upper body from hips—drop head—turn hips to left, circling chi ball over the head to the right side—shift tailbone to right heel.

28. Brush Knee: Step left heel back to south—turn right foot 45 degrees west—drop left hand brushing left knee—shift tailbone to center—push right hand forward.

◎ *Fourth Round, Facing Southeast: Left-Hand Form*

29. SE Corner: Bird's Tail to north—Single Whip to southeast—Flying Oblique, Lift Hand Step Forward, and White Crane facing east—Brush Knee strike to southeast–change directions 180 degrees.

◎ *Fifth Round, Facing Northwest: Right-Hand Form*

30. NW Corner: Bird's Tail to southeast—Single Whip to northeast–Flying Oblique, Lift Hand Step Forward, and White Crane facing east—Brush Knee strike to northwest—change directions 135 degrees.

◎ *Sixth Round, Facing Southwest: Left-Hand Form*

31. SW Corner: Bird's Tail to northwest—Single Whip to northeast—Flying Oblique, Lift Hand Step Forward, and White Crane facing

north—Brush Knee strike to southwest—change directions 180 degrees.

❃ Seventh Round, Facing Northeast: Right-Hand Form

32. NE Corner: Bird's Tail strike to southwest—Single Whip to southeast—Flying Oblique, Lift Hand Step Forward, and White Crane facing south—Brush Knee strike to northeast—change directions 45 degrees.

❃ Closing the Form

1. Completion: Shift tailbone to right hip and release transition. Open both hands, moving them up, outward, and downward. Draw left foot straight back, setting it down next to the right foot. Shift tailbone to the left heel and lift up the right leg, placing it parallel with the left. Draw feet together with toes even.

2. Cross Hands: Raise hands 12 inches in front of body to form an X below the shoulders, with the left hand closer to the body.

3. Distribute weight evenly between both feet. Simultaneously straighten body and lower hands to sides with palms facing back. End all movements at the same time.

4. Relax and center yourself; feel the chi expand in your body.

5. Smile down and collect energy at the navel.

Pages 153 to 168 provide an easy visual guide for your daily Tai Chi Chi Kung Wu Style practice.

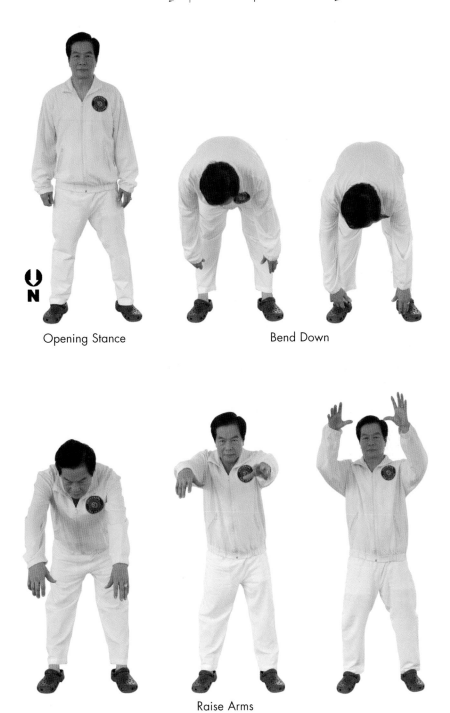

Opening Stance   Bend Down

Raise Arms

Fig. 6.1. Opening the form

Opening Movements

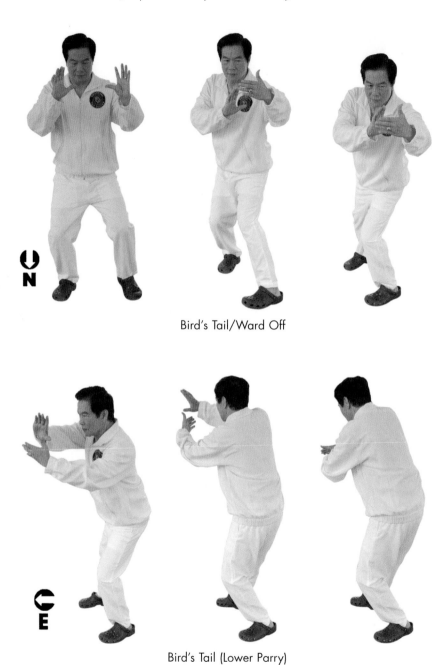

Bird's Tail/Ward Off

Bird's Tail (Lower Parry)

Fig. 6.2. Bird's Tail (to east)

Core Movements: Right-Hand Form (Facing North)

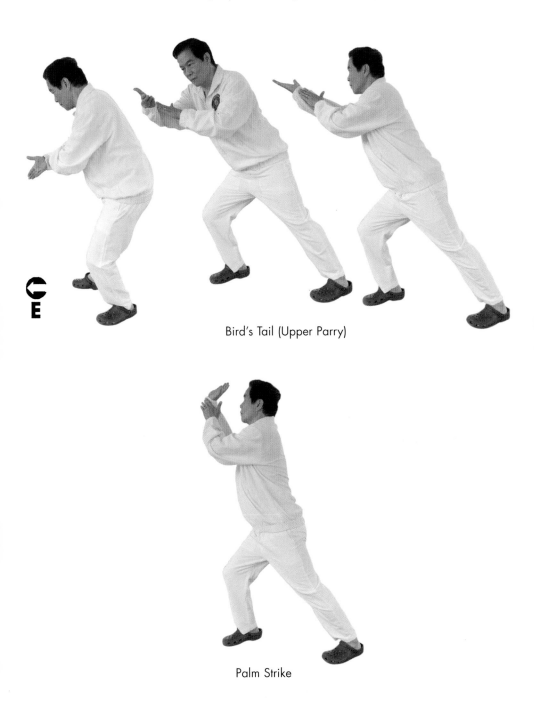

Bird's Tail (Upper Parry)

Palm Strike

Fig. 6.3. End of Bird's Tail with Palm Strike

Core Movements: Right-Hand Form (Facing North)

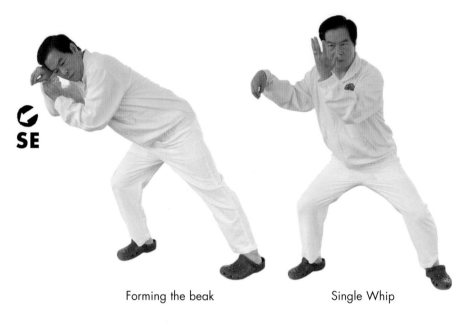

Forming the beak   Single Whip

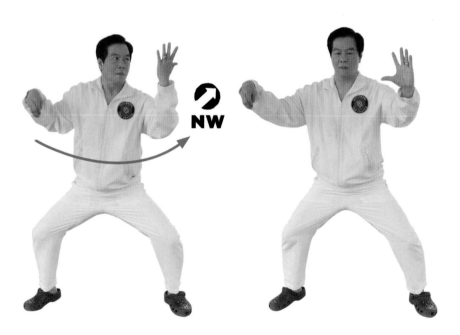

Single Whip, continued

Fig. 6.4. Single Whip (to northwest)

Core Movements: Right-Hand Form (Facing North)

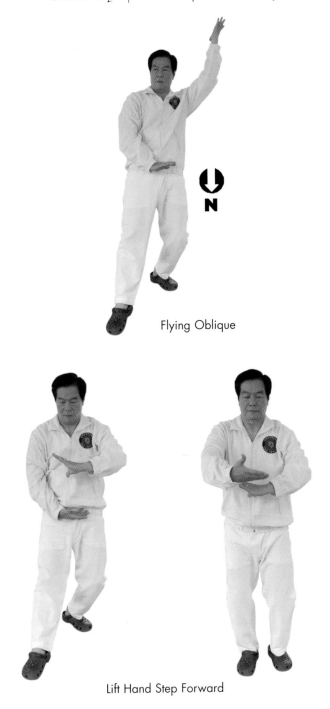

Flying Oblique

Lift Hand Step Forward

Fig. 6.5. Flying Oblique and Lift Hand Step Forward (to north)

Core Movements: Right-Hand Form (Facing North)

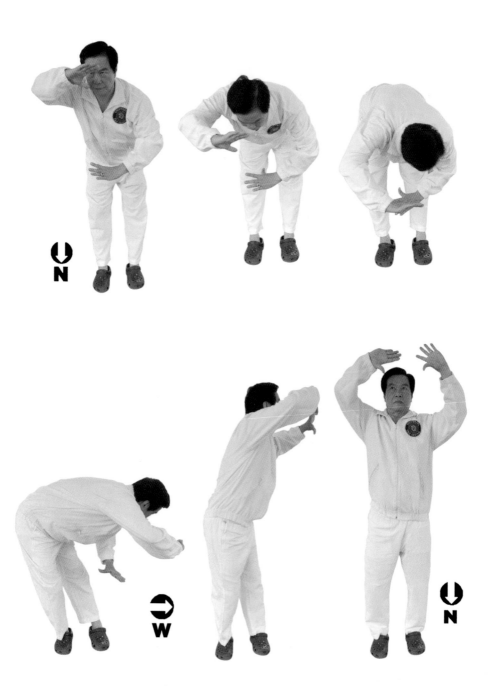

Fig. 6.6. White Crane Spreads Its Wings (to north)

Core Movements: Right-Hand Form (Facing North)

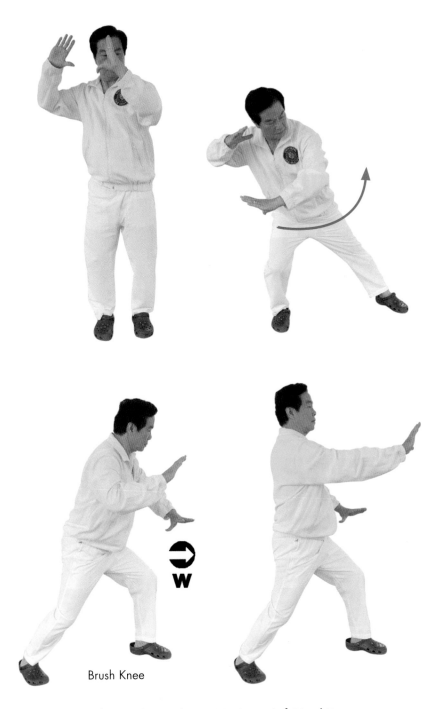

Brush Knee

Fig. 6.7. Brush Knee (to west), transitioning to Left-Hand Form to west

Core Movements: Right-Hand Form (Facing North)

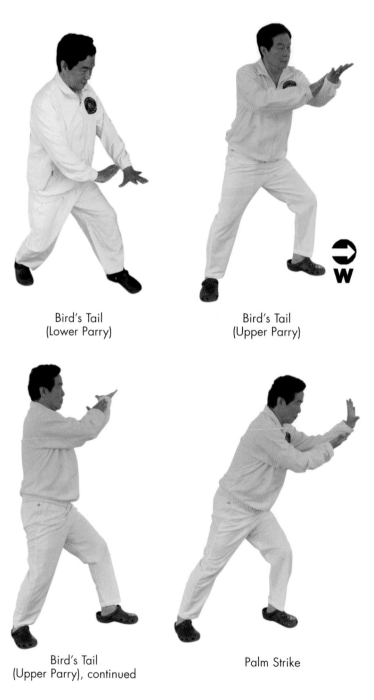

Bird's Tail
(Lower Parry)

Bird's Tail
(Upper Parry)

Bird's Tail
(Upper Parry), continued

Palm Strike

Fig. 6.8. Bird's Tail (to west)

Core Movements: Left-Hand Form (Facing West)

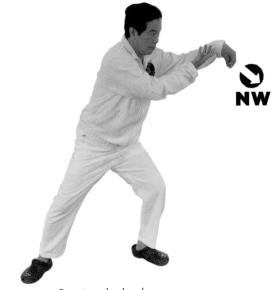

Forming the beak
in the northwest

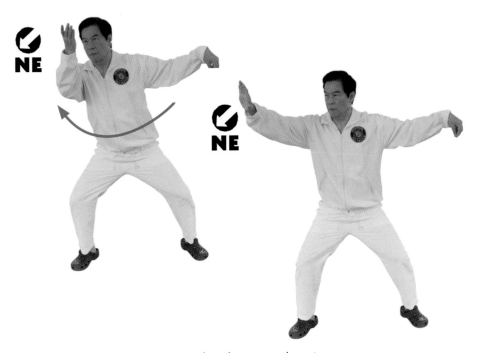

Fig. 6.9. Single Whip (to northeast)

Core Movements: Left-Hand Form (Facing West)

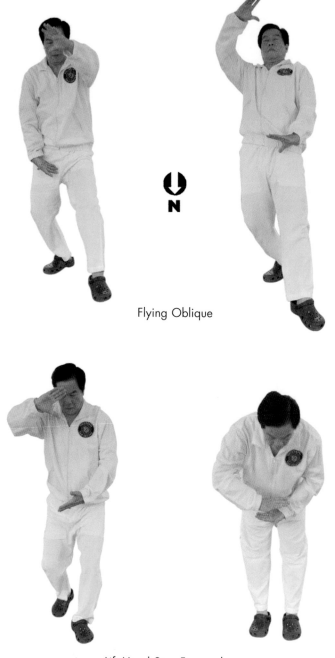

Flying Oblique

Lift Hand Step Forward

Fig. 6.10. Flying Oblique and Lift Hand Step Forward (to north)

Core Movements: Left-Hand Form (Facing West)

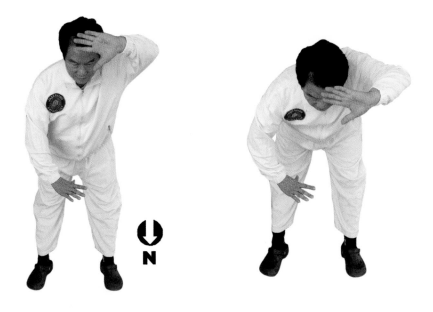

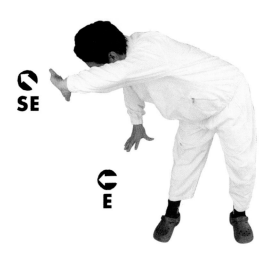

Fig. 6.11. White Crane Spreads Its Wings (to north)

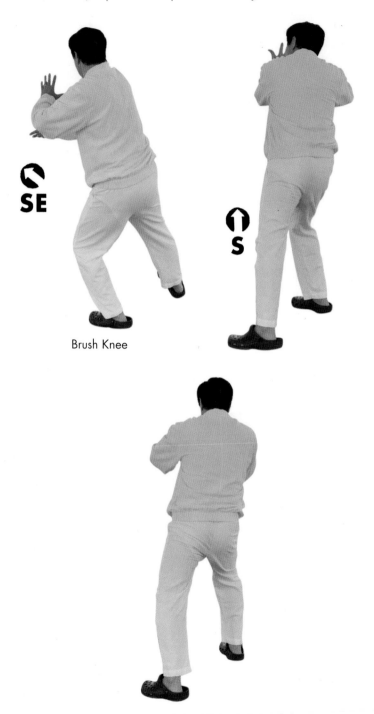

Brush Knee

Fig. 6.12. Brush Knee and transition to Right-Hand Form to south

Core Movements: Right-Hand Form (Facing South)

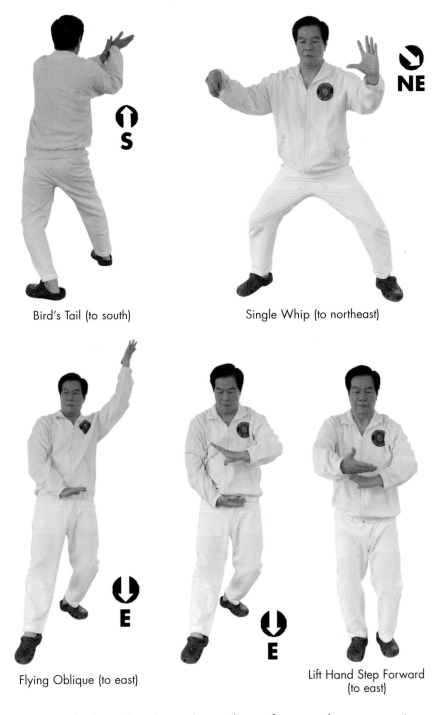

Bird's Tail (to south)

Single Whip (to northeast)

Flying Oblique (to east)

Lift Hand Step Forward (to east)

Fig. 6.13. Third round, Right-Hand Form (begins facing south, turns to east)

Core Movements: Right-Hand Form (Facing South)

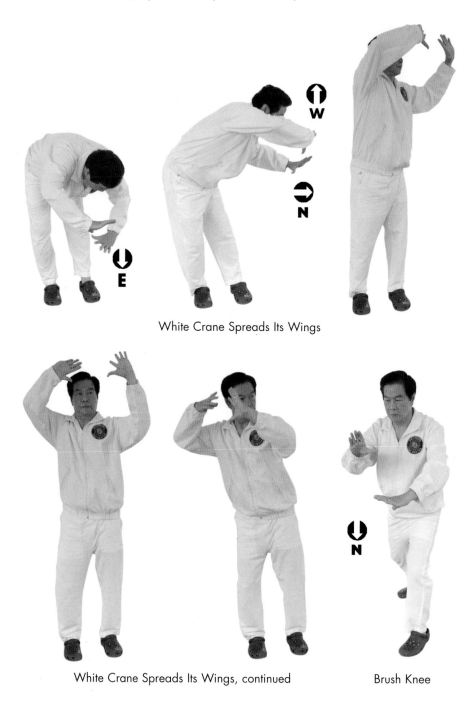

White Crane Spreads Its Wings

White Crane Spreads Its Wings, continued

Brush Knee

Fig. 6.14. White Crane Spreads Its Wings (to east) and Brush Knee (to north)

Core Movements: Right-Hand Form (Facing South)

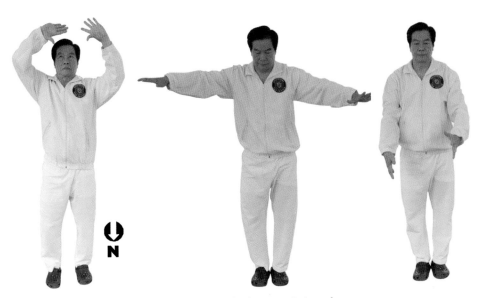

Bring hands down and close feet

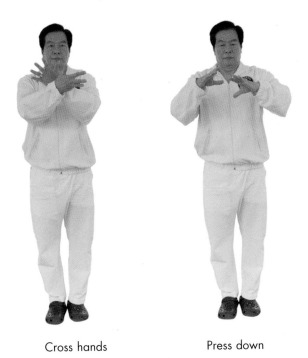

Cross hands   Press down

Fig. 6.15. Closing the form

Closing Form

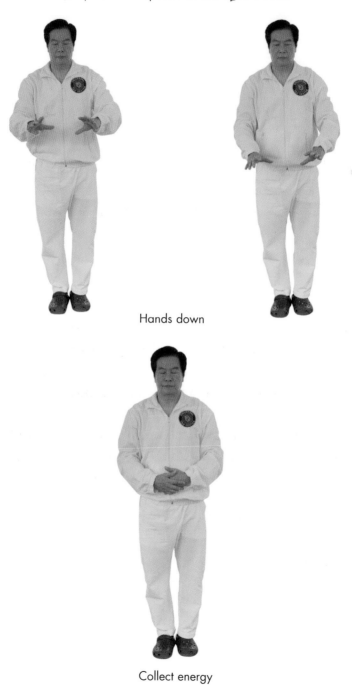

Hands down

Collect energy

Fig. 6.15. Closing the form, continued

Closing Form

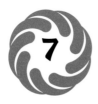

Martial Applications of the Wu Style Form

The Wu Style Form will look its best to onlookers if it is performed with the inherent meaning of the martial art moves—otherwise, it can look like a purposeless waving of the arms. The only way to understand the martial applications is to spend time practicing them with a partner.

On first inspection, the short form may appear simple, with one application per form. However, on deeper examination there are many more applications. This chapter will break down the short form and explain the meanings of the postures and individual forms. Sources for the applications were drawn from both the Southern and Northern schools. In the Southern school, they were inspired by teachers such as Chen Tin-Hung, Rocky Kwong, and John Yuen. In the Northern school they were learned from Liu Hong-Chi as part of Li Bing-Ci's 45-posture competition Wu form, with some references to Wang Pei-Sheng's text on the 37-posture Wu style.

Opening Form

Although it is not seen in many Wu forms,* the Universal Healing Tao Forward Bend at the commencement of the form can be applied

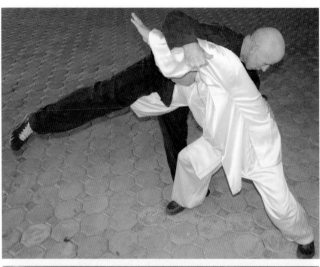

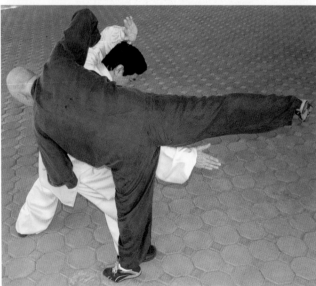

Fig. 7.1. Forward bend with shoulder throw and high attack dodge

---

*For instance, the Bend Down form is not found in: Wang Pei-Sheng's 37 form, Cheng Tin Hung's long form, Wu Kam-Chin's 119 long form or the Northern style long or competition form of Li Bing-Ci.

to many combat situations. The most obvious application is a dodge for a high attack (fig. 7.1). This occurs when an opponent's center of gravity is high with a forward-moving momentum. The practitioner gets underneath the opponent's center and follows the opponent's forward momentum with a high shoulder throw. Alternatively, it can be a response to finding oneself under the arms of the opponent.

The opening form can be described as including the four major forces or Gates of Peng, Lu, Ji, and An. These will be explained shortly within the applications of this beginning form.

The forward bend includes rising arms, which involves a Peng force. This force can be applied to the opponent's arms when in a stranglehold or lock (fig. 7.2). Peng means that the power is amplified from the earth and that it is loaded in the tan tien like a coiled spring. The rising arms can strike the elbows or forearms, releasing the lock.

The contact with the opponent's arms is akin to the Ji force. In

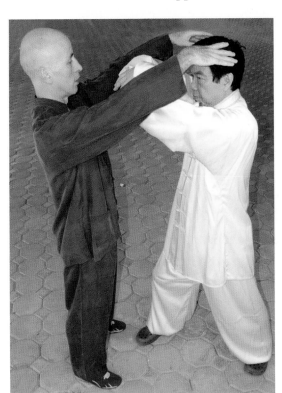

Fig. 7.2. Peng force releasing a strangle

*Tai Chi Fa Jin,** the Ji force was explained using the Press as its outward gross manifestation. However, in a more subtle interpretation it can be understood as the power from a rubbing force in close contact. From this rubbing close contact, the opponent can be uprooted using the tan tien force (fig. 7.3); this interaction is visualized as a coin bouncing off a drum.

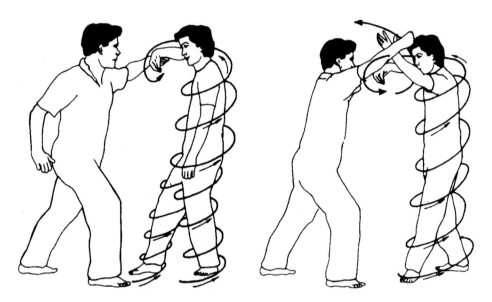

Fig. 7.3. Using Ji force to uproot an opponent

From the strike with the rising arms, the arms can fall—grabbing the arms of the opponent in the process and pulling him down (fig. 7.4). As the hands return to the lower tan tien, they contain the Lu force or the power of emptiness. The last component of this form is an An force, which executes a pushing or striking force at the last moment. So the final gesture of this Pull Down can be throwing the opponent.

---

*See *Tai Chi Fa Jin* (Rochester, Vt.: Destiny Books, 2012).

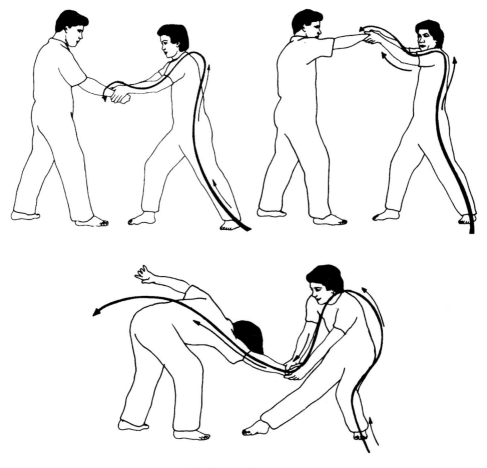

Fig. 7.4. Pull Down

 Bird's Tail

Many applications can arise during the various components of the Bird's Tail. Below, the Bird's Tail form is broken down into its component parts, and each part's applications are explored.

⊙ *Ward Off*

The Forward Ward Off is the first component of the Bird's Tail (fig. 7.5); it occurs with the right arm and leg forward. There are several applications of the Ward Off.

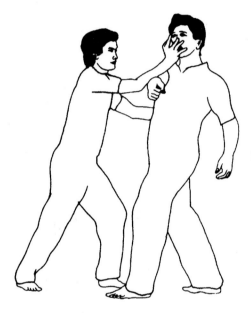

Fig. 7.5. Ward Off

The first application is a hip throw, whereby the rear arm is placed on the chest, the front arm placed behind the opponent, and the hip or front leg are placed behind the opponent to topple him. Alternatively, the Ward Off can be used as a strike/block with the rear hand acting as a secondary guard.

An Elbow Strike can be inserted after the Ward Off and before the lower hand rotation (fig. 7.6). Some may argue that this is over-reaching the form, but it is important to realize how many different forms can arise from simple discharge movements of the tan tien. The outward manifestations of the eight forces can appear from seemingly nothing, crystallizing as applications from formless water. For this move, the elbow or Chou Gate can be used.

From the right Ward Off the hands transit through the Seven Stars (Play the Pi Pa) position (see fig. 7.7 on page 176). The Seven

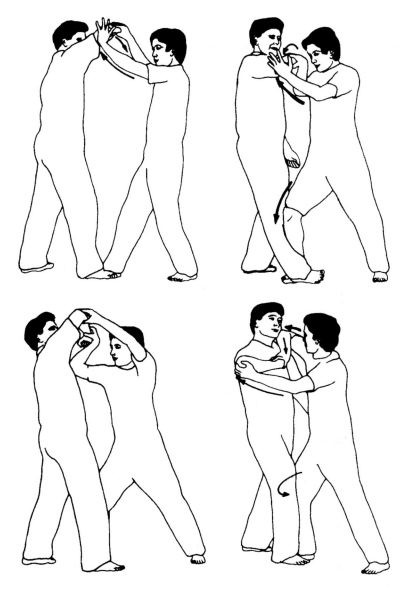

Fig. 7.6. Elbow Strike

Stars can be used to trap a strike by controlling the elbow and thereby breaking the opponent's Iron Shirt posture. The arms are released centrally from this position to execute a one-inch strike with the front arm while the rear arm imparts jin to the trapped elbow. Once the

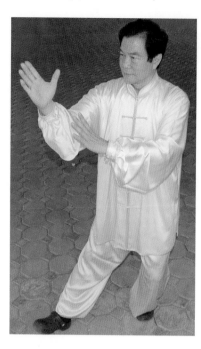

Fig. 7.7. Seven Stars
(Play the Pi Pa) position

structure is broken, any attack is possible. A second application is a static one, whereby the arms merely move into a front guard position.

Lower Parry

In the Downward Parry the novice practitioner would focus on the hands. However, to the experienced adept, much is concealed in this seemingly simple rotation of the waist with the palms downward. The left shoulder can be used from the posterior position to create a shoulder or Kou strike as the adept rotates the waist (fig. 7.8).

This application raises an important fundamental principle of Tai Chi Boxing. All outward gates or applications can arise from simple rotations of the waist and expansive discharge from the lower tan tien. There are three basic discharges possible from the force created in the tan tien—an upward, downward, or angular discharge. The part of the body that ends up using the force is only a minor consideration. Simplicity is the key to accessing true power in this internal art: from it a detailed armory of techniques can arise. Continue to ask yourself what

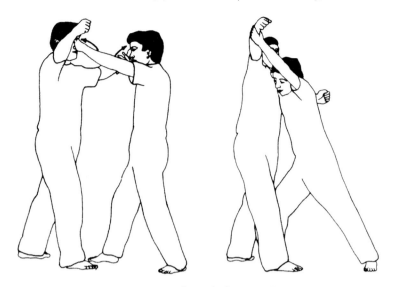

Fig. 7.8. Kou strike with the rear shoulder

is the simple power under each move and eventually you will learn the fundamentals of Tai Chi.

Of course, the Lower Arm Sweep can be used as a Lower Parry or block, as shown below (fig. 7.9). Being aware of the myriad outward

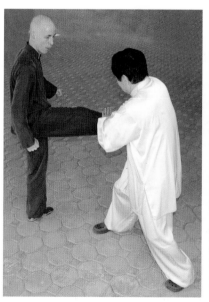
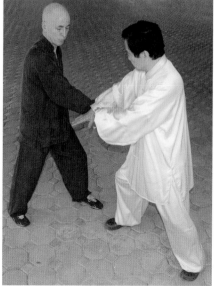

Fig. 7.9. Lower Arm Sweep

manifestations of each posture brings out the true spirit of the form. It also keeps the primary trunk and core strength of the lower tan tien active and ready to release its power at the blink of an eye.

⟳ Upper Arm Parry

In the Upper Arm Parry of the Bird's Tail, there are several applications. The first is an upper block for a strike—usually a Roundhouse Punch—in which the adept finds himself face to face with the opponent (fig. 7.10). Note that the ideal position is to encounter the opponent to one side, which restricts the number of strikes that the adept can receive. However, there will always be times when the adept comes face to face with an opponent; this will be discussed in further detail in the next chapter.

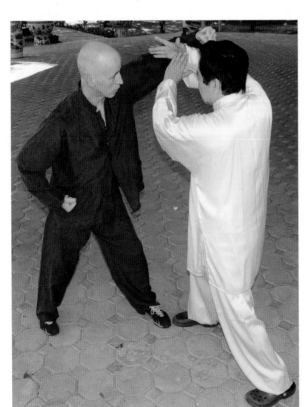

Fig. 7.10. Upper Arm Parry

A second application is like an upward-directed Press (fig. 7.11). In this scenario the opponent can be directed upward and backward using the Ji Gate.

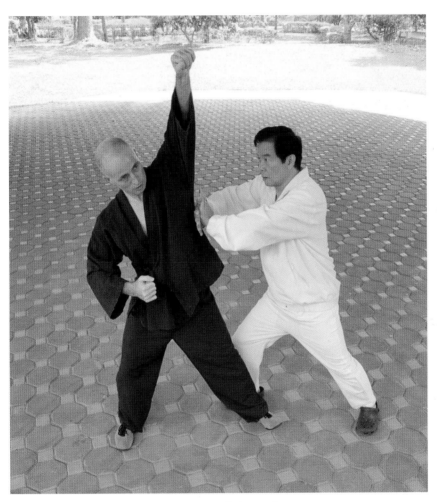

Fig. 7.11. Upward-directed Press

Push

The application of the right-hand Angled (Forward) Push of the Bird's Tail is reasonably straightforward. It is a simple strike with the palm initially led by the hypothenar eminence or the ulnar aspect of the palm (fig. 7.12). As will be discussed in the next chapter, the accomplished practitioner moves away from literal interpretations of the applications to an integrated understanding. A form only has power in the setting of a complex sequence of moves against an opponent who is responding to the adept's moves. When the opponent withdraws the adept will advance. The power lies in the complimenting of another's moves. There is no power in isolation.

This move can also be incorporated as part of the Wu Boxing's repertoire of the Bird's Tail. As one follows the returning vector of an opponent's Roundhouse Punch, the hand effortlessly strikes. This can be an open palm as in the form or a fist. In the final instant the An Gate is used.

Single Whip

One application of the Single Whip is to grab a wrist and take your arm under the opponent's elbow for a throw backward over your knee. A second application is to grab the wrist and strike the same elbow or shoulder that corresponds to the opponent's wrist. A third application is to use the Single Whip with the Lieh force and deliver a simultaneous trap and strike (see fig. 7.13 on page 182).

Flying Oblique

In the Wu style, the spine is slanted and the elbow on the upward arm is at more of an acute angle. The focus can then be put on the shoulder, allowing this form to represent the implementation of the Kou Force (see fig. 7.14 on page 182).

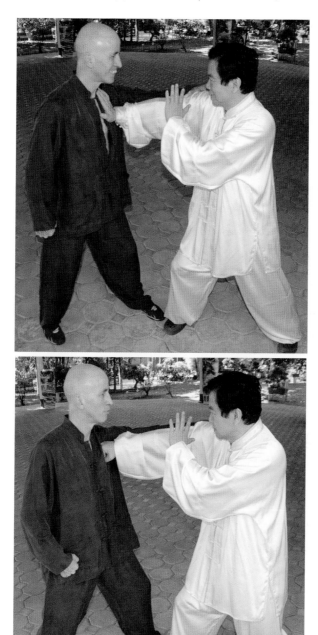

Fig. 7.12. Hand Angled (Forward) Push

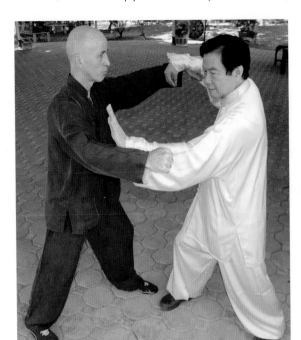

Fig. 7.13. Single Whip

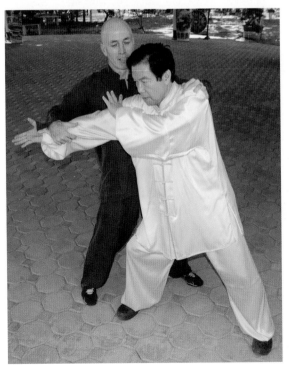

Fig. 7.14. Flying Oblique

Lift Hand and Step Forward

This form has two moves. The first is a Press and the second is an Upward Strike or Parry (fig. 7.15). The Press can be initiated in a couple of ways. In Push Hands it is often performed after an opponent's Push, which is diverted to the side using the Lu Gate. This exposes the shoulder or ribs, which can then be attacked using the Press with the Ji force.

Wang Pei-Sheng likes to initiate this move with a lock (Tsoi Gate) to the opponent's forearm. The straightening of the elbow breaks the Iron Shirt structure and therefore invites a withdrawal response, against which the Press (Ji Gate) can be used (see fig. 7.16 on page 184).[1]

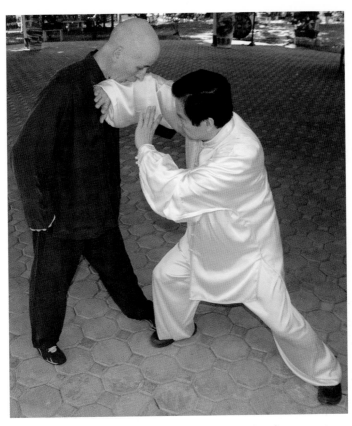

Fig. 7.15. Lift Hand and Step Forward

The Lift Hand component of this form can be used either as a strike or an Upward Parry with the hand or the forearm (fig. 7.17).

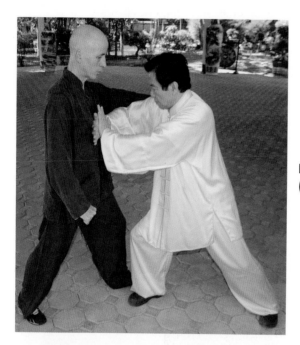

Fig. 7.16. Press (Ji Gate)

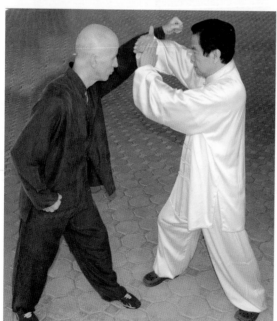

Fig. 7.17. Strike or Upward Parry

White Crane Spreads Its Wings

This form shows some of the unique characteristics of the Wu style. The more extensive and elaborate circles emphasize its flowing rounds, which originate in the waist and create a pattern akin to the art of calligraphy. This complex move includes a dodge, then an entry with the application of a lock/throw using the Tsoi gate (fig. 7.19).

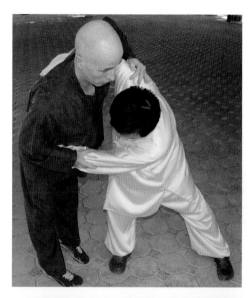

Fig. 7.18. White Crane Spreads Its Wings

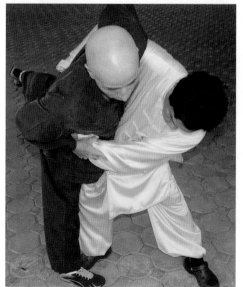

Fig. 7.19. Hip throw using the Tsoi gate

Brush Knee

This form includes a parry followed by a Palm Strike with one hand and a Lower Block with the other (fig. 7.20). The first parry is known in the Wu style as the Cross Hands. In this application a head high strike by the opponent is gently guided to the side. In the more complex version cited in the next chapter, both hands engage in a block instead of just one. The block then creates entry for a Palm Strike.

Unique to the Wu system is the slanting spine, which, as discussed in the introductory chapters, allows several extra phenomena

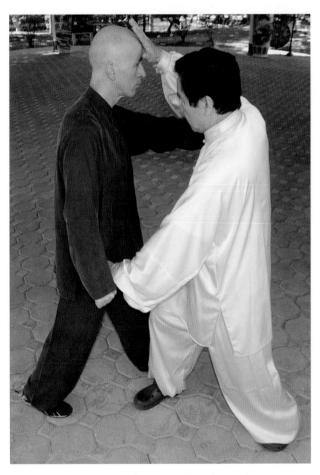

Fig. 7.20. Brush Knee with Palm Strike

to occur. The first is that it is easier to allow the jin to rise from the earth through the legs and up the spine without impediment. This manifests physically as a tucking of the coccyx, reduction of the lumbar lordosis, widening of the scapulae, and tucking in of the chin. In other words, the whole body is rooted and forms a preparatory Iron Shirt for the moment of impact. Secondly, the strike can transmit a downward vector of the body weight as well, transferring all of the adept's body weight to the opponent. This creates the potential for a very damaging blow.

The Lower Parry can be used at the same time to block a strike originating from the opponent's arm or leg.

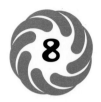

The Wu Style Tai Chi Boxing System

We believe the Wu style has embraced a most effective boxing system. Whereas the Chen boxing style is strong, powerful, and martial in outward appearance, overtly displaying Fa Jin, it demonstrates fighting in fragments within individual applications, rather than a coherent fighting system. Similarly, the Yang style has health benefits, but also demonstrates Fa Jin separately from the long form. The Southern Wu system, in contrast, has a legitimate, systematized, and effective boxing system.*

As discussed in chapter 1, the origin of the fighting system is in some doubt. The boxing system that we are going to share in this chapter comes from the lineage of Chen Tin-Hung. Master Chen changed the name of his form from Wu style to Wu Tang style because of his amalgamation of Wu style with an internal style fighting system from the Wu Tang Mountain. It is obvious that Chen Tin-Hung's long form is the Wu style; it is also obvious that the boxing system is based on the long form. However, as the reader will realize,

---

*The Wu boxing system has proven its effectiveness: in 1980, Dan Docherty (a student of Chen Tin-Hung) used Wu Tai Chi Boxing and won the Open Weight Division of the Fifth South East Asian Chinese Pugilistic Championships in Malaysia.

the boxing system is more than just segments of the long form sped up; it has peculiarities and themes of its own. Most of the themes are based on Push Hands theory and the deeper principles of Taoism.

It is important to remember that styles of martial arts are fluid and involved in an ever-changing process. Fundamentalists would say that a style should always be corrected in alignment with the original master's methods. Innovators would hold the opposite view—that each style or master has practices that can be improved upon or modified to suit new environments. Wu Chuan-Yu changed the original (Yang) form and practices as did Wu Yu-Hsiang, who modified the Yang to the Hao style, and Sun Lu-Tang, who drew on the Hao and Wu styles to create the Sun style. Of course, changing forms and practices must come from a well-considered space and not simply from laziness or lack of skill.

In a sense, each practitioner constructs something new, infusing prior knowledge and frameworks with new information to arrive at a system that is truly her own. Of course, it takes a Grand Master's capabilities to create a whole new system, but the constructivist principles can be seen in many levels of practice.

With this in mind, it is important to remember that the system presented in this book is different from the ones taught by Eddie Yee, Chen Tin-Hung, Kwong Ken-Yue, or John Yuen—and their masters before them. We respect and honor the teachers listed above, and trust that a special and enduring thread remains between their teachings and ours. Perhaps we can go as far as to suggest that deficiencies in one generation may be remedied by generations later; perhaps teaching methods need to change to suit the learning needs of current generations. In any case, it is through the virtues of faith and hope that such wondrous Taoist arts can endure and influence mankind in a positive way.

With the above preamble in mind, we will emphasize the following themes in this chapter. First, this system is unique in its adherence to the principles of Push Hands. Second, and ever pervasive, is the relationship of this pugilistic art with the philosophy of the Tao, which manifests with a return to the simple and natural. Third, the postures themselves are kept high with a narrow stance, while movements incorporate natural protective reflexes. Fourth, postures are made conducive to the generation of power from the lower tan tien.

Ideally, a practitioner learning the boxing system will already have studied Iron Shirt training, Tan Tien Chi Kung, the short Yang form, the short Wu form, and the Yang Discharge Form. A long Wu form is also helpful, but not essential.

SOUTHERN WU BOXING SYSTEM

The Wu Tai Chi Boxing system can best be described by first outlining the basic strikes and parries. From these basic steps, the more complex forms—which have been modified from the short and long forms to suit actual fighting scenarios—can then be studied. Remember that the slow form has a different purpose. While it helps students develop a healing integration of body, mind, chi, and jin within the framework of martial moves, these fundamentals are assumed in the actual applications, which must be performed with an opponent at fast speeds. Now, injury to the opponent becomes an objective. In other words, the boxing applications are not merely segments of the form sped up; they require a new set of themes and rules to enable transplantation from the slow form to the fighting arena.

The trouble with boxing is that opponents fight back. This necessitates the incorporation of moves that protect the adept from strikes. In addition, each move must be located in space and time so as to take advantage of the opponent's strikes and the anatomy of his or her limbs. The principles of Push Hands are applied in all situations, which means that practitioners strive to obtain physical contact as much as possible. Therefore, the perception, detection, and interpretation of an opponent's moves have to breach a more refined level. An opponent's spirit is interpreted by the adept's mind taking in clues from visual, tactile, and energetic phenomena. Because the adept has turned on his integrated mind, awareness is now possible outside the body—even with the eyes closed. The practitioner can perceive the opponent's chi, jin, and intentions.

The range of boxing moves is purposely limited. A practitioner of average capability can simply learn the basic moves of Palm Strike, Punching, and Back Fist, and the more complex moves of Cross Hands, Bird's Tail, Willow Tree, Closing the Gate, and Single Whip. Having a small repertoire of moves that are totally familiar is better than knowing a vast range of techniques that are only moderately understood. In the words of Master John Yuen, "It is better to have a few sharp knives than a thousand blunt ones." Nevertheless, there are occasional times when the adept calls upon peripheral techniques such as the Lotus Kick or Snake Creeps Down. A brief description of other applications occurs in chapter 7.

THE BASIC MOVES

The fundamental moves that we cover here include the Palm Strike, Punching, and Back Fist; combination moves like Back Fist and Punch, and Double Strikes; variant punches like Roundhouse and Uppercut; and Parries.

The Palm Strike

The Palm Strike is used frequently in Tai Chi Chuan and its boxing applications. It is found in the short form in Grasping the Bird's Tail and Brush Knee forms, and in the long form in Pat the High Horse, Repulse Monkey, Fan through the Back, Fair Lady Works the Shuttle, and Palm Strike to the Face. The uniqueness of the Palm Strike in the Wu style has already been mentioned earlier in this text: because the stance is shorter and the spine is slanted, a downward component vector can enter into this strike (see fig. 8.1 on page 192). With a straight spine, power or jin is obligated only to have a horizontal component, and the heel of the palm must be emphasized. In the Wu style, the adept can add a downward vector by bending the knees and dropping the whole body to the ground at the moment of impact.

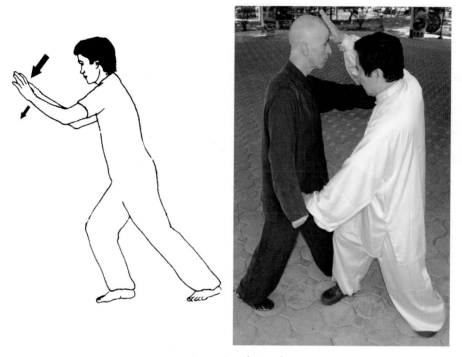

Fig. 8.1. Palm Strike

Punching

Although it does not appear in the Universal Healing Tao Wu Style Short Form, punching is a vital part of the boxing system. It is used in the long Wu form within the following forms: Parry and Punch, Fist Under Elbow, Punch Down, Punch Low, Boxing the Ears, Fight Tiger, Draw the Bow, and Shoot the Tiger.

The Wu style punch is different from karate and other punches in several respects. First, the Wu punch strikes with the outer three knuckles (ulnar side) instead of the inner knuckles (radial side). Because force is transmitted best via the curved and spiral structure of the Iron Shirt rather than a straight line, the wrist must be slightly deviated toward the radius (fig. 8.2). Otherwise, the force of impact would be transmitted to the wrists rather than up the arm. Remember that in accordance with Iron Shirt principles, force

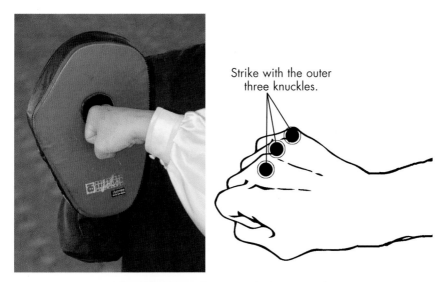

Strike with the outer
three knuckles.

Fig. 8.2. Wrist alignment during a punch

is transmitted from the earth through the legs, the spine, and out through the shoulder girdle. Power and force are best transmitted when all muscles and tendons are relaxed to length.

Another unique aspect of Wu Style Boxing is that the punch originates from the Central Thrusting Channel at the level of the heart (see fig. 8.3 on page 194). In Western boxing or karate, by contrast, the punch originates from a position to the side of the central axis. Having a central axis means that for both sides, the vector of power originates from the same point; this centralization protects the midline. While a Western boxer might argue that there could be some loss of power by originating the punch from the midline, for a Wu style practitioner, the principle of maintaining one's center outweighs any possible reduction in external power.

Multiple punches create a circular pattern. Each punch drops down after reaching its full length and returns underneath the next outgoing punch. The direction of the punches can change from left to right, high to low, and even alternate from one aspect to another with single punches and yet still keep circling around the same central focal point.

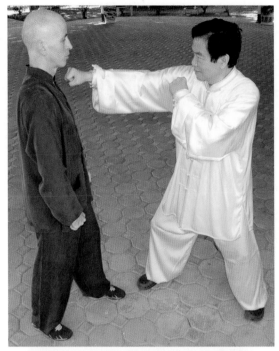

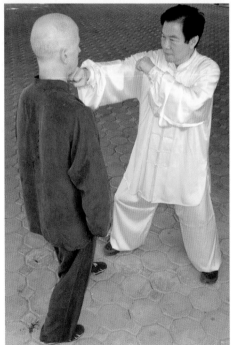

Fig. 8.3. Punch from the central axis.

⟳ *Punching Technical Exercise*

Punch for one to three minutes with a partner who varies the height and horizontal placement of the mitt.

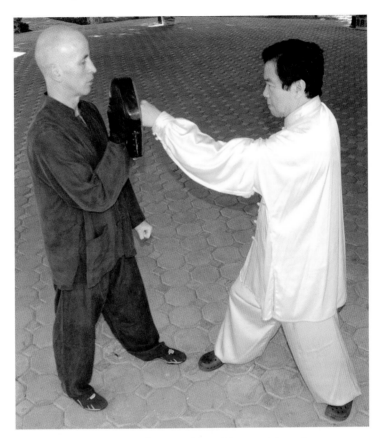

Fig. 8.4. Punching partner with protective mitt

An Introduction to the Discharge Principles of Strikes

A simple fist strike follows all the principles of discharge power. First, the body must be loose and relaxed: the purpose is to use jin rather than external li power. Second, the recoil is just as important as the strike itself, just like in the slow form. The recoil is directed by the chi and the empty force, which then activates the structure. Chi or jin is stored for a moment in the earth, then we rotate the waist and jin passes up through the legs, pelvis, spine, and arm (fig. 8.5). The jin is like a wave that explodes in the earth and travels longitudinally (fig. 8.6).

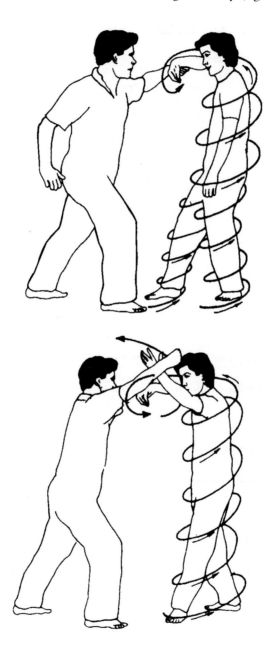

Fig. 8.5. Activation of jin (yin phase)

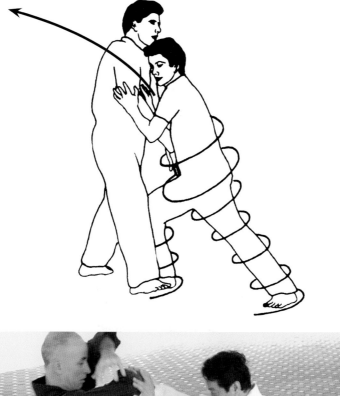

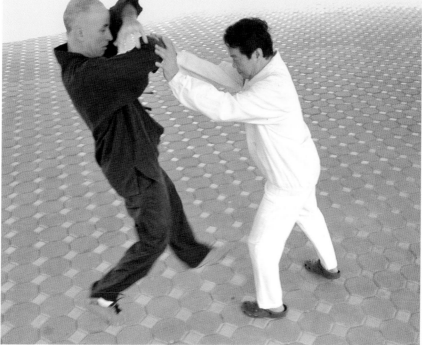

Fig. 8.6. Jin passing through the structure (yang phase)

In fast speed the principle is the same. The recoil will entail either sticking to or following an opponent's intended strike; the recoil then sets up the discharge. Although the practitioner remains still on the outside, activation of the internal structure and jin still occurs on the inside.

 ## Back Fist

Back Fist is a part of most Wu long forms, though it does not appear in the Universal Healing Tao Short Wu Form. With practice, the principles of transmission of power remain the same whether one strikes with the palm, knuckles, elbow, or back fist. The choice of the final contact or weapon depends on circumstance. A Back Fist arises when the practitioner is at an acute angle to the opponent and the hands are near the hip (fig. 8.7). The jin power is easily activated, and time is saved as the practitoner avoids withdrawing the arm and repositioning it. A Back Fist can be part of a flurry of strikes, because any strike can metamorphose into any form on its circular return.

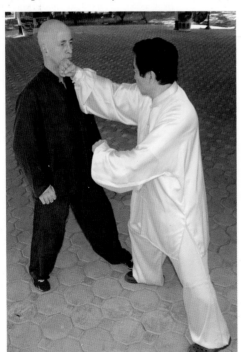

Fig. 8.7. Back Fist showing upward and horizontal arc vector

Internal Discharge Power Principles of the Back Fist

The strike power for the Back Fist comes from the earth through the legs and finally a rotation of the tan tien. The vector of force is both upward and horizontal. The striking point is the back of the fist (dorsum of the hand).

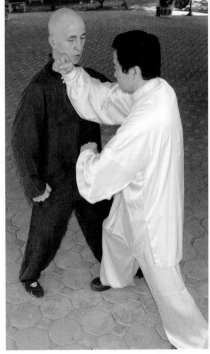 Double Strikes

Double strikes make use of the power that is generated by one core movement—a flick of the tan tien. What is placed on the end of this core is variable and can include diverse anatomical weapons and also multiple strikes. The double strike can include a combination of Back Fist and a Punch (fig. 8.8), or a Back Fist and a Palm Strike, or just a Double Punch. The core movement generates the power, while the

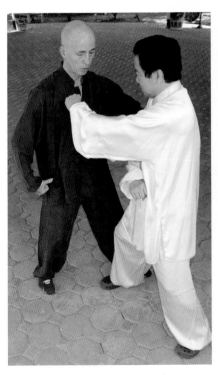

Fig. 8.8. Flick of the waist, with Punch and Back Fist

strike takes the shape that is suited to the interaction between adept and opponent at that particular moment.

 ## Variant Punches: Roundhouse and Uppercut

Variant punches include the Roundhouse Punch (fig. 8.9) and the Uppercut. The Roundhouse Punch is used in the long form during Fight Tiger, Draw the Bow to Shoot the Tiger, and Boxing the Ears. The Uppercut is used in Fist under the Elbow. The spirit of punches is often associated with the tiger; when we imagine fighting like a tiger our eyes open, unnecessary tension is reduced, and power increases.

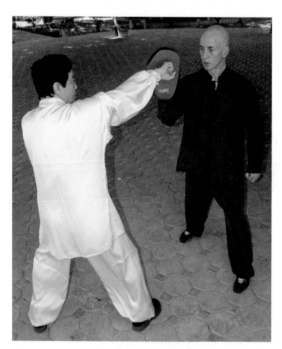

Fig. 8.9. Roundhouse Punch (with protective mitt)

 ## Parries

Parries are found in the Universal Healing Tao Short Form as part of the Brush Knee and Bird's Tail forms. They can range from single palm deflections to multiple continuous circular parries; they can involve either the backs (dorsum) or the palms of the hands, or a combination of both (fig. 8.10). At the highest level, it is difficult to distinguish a parry from a strike. The hand motions combine into

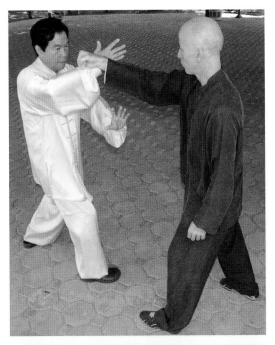

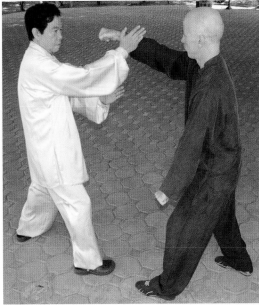

Fig. 8.10. Circular parries using the dorsum, then palm, of the hand

circular movements that spiral clockwise or counterclockwise from shoulder to hip. It is this continuous spiraling that gave rise to the name silk reeling for these exercises. From a Taoist mystical perspective, the spirals mimic the effortless cosmic dance of all energetic phenomena.

🌀 Deeper Jin Principles of Parries

Parries in Tai Chi Boxing are different from those found in many martial arts. They are not intended to significantly deflect or injure; instead, they are a means of engaging with an opponent at close range. Such contact enables the skills of ting and dong jin (listening and understanding jin), which will have a significant impact on the adept. From an attitude of aggression and maximum deflection, the adept will move to a space of calm observation with the intention to follow and join. This takes fear out of the equation, and the adept finds himself more successful at negating strikes. Furthermore, from this intention to follow and join, the eight forces can be activated. The parries draw the opponent in as close as possible without causing injury to the practitioner. Remaining close and connected is the theme.

The silk-reeling exercises and applications discussed in *Tai Chi Fa Jin** can be converted into parries on either the back of the hand or the palmar sides. The beauty of the Wu style and its round form (such as that displayed by Chen Tin-Hung) is its emphasis on ongoing circular parries. These parries can manage a barrage of strikes due to their circular base; they can easily change external shape to the more complex patterns (like Cross Hands, Bird's Tail, Willow Tree, and Closing the Gate) without interruption.

---

*See pp. 92–93 and 98–101 in *Tai Chi Fa Jin* (Rochester, Vt.: Destiny Books, 2012).

COMPLEX BOXING FORMS

The complex forms of Wu style boxing include the Bird's Tail, Cross Hands, Willow Tree, Close the Gate, and the Single Whip.

Bird's Tail

The boxing application of the Bird's Tail uses the same sequence as the short form. As mentioned in chapter 5, the spirit of this move is likened to grasping a wagging bird's tail. An opponent's strikes occur in a flurry and dart here and there. The aim is to both avoid these and execute an injuring strike. The Bird's Tail is comprised of a circular Upward Parry with one forearm while the other palm uses a splitting force—as a counterbalance and a simultaneous block or strike. This double move is then followed by a double strike (usually straight punches).

Deeper Push Hands Principles of the Bird's Tail

The initial arm block is usually used against a Roundhouse Punch: the power of the opponent is used to convert this parry into an injuring strike. A round punch by its nature must eventually have a vector of force that returns to itself. The initial parry of this move takes advantage of this vector and rides it toward its origin. Thus the power of the Bird's Tail's ultimate strike is doubled—the jin of the adept is added to the borrowed power of the opponent. Furthermore, since the opponent is pulling his arm back toward himself, he cannot retaliate. No space or time is allowed for him to retract and strike again. The simultaneous split or strike that occurs with this Upward Parry is used primarily to negate any possible counterstrike that the opponent might initiate. The strike uses a Tiger Palm, which jams the inside of the elbow (see fig. 8.11 on page 204).

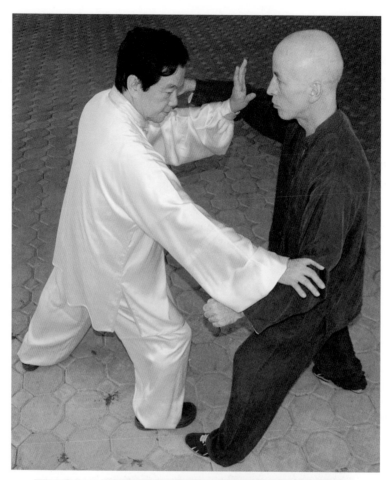

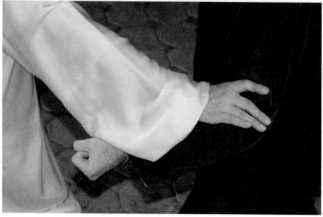

Fig. 8.11. Tiger Palm for
jamming the elbow

❂ *Ideal Position for the Bird's Tail Form*

The ideal position for the Bird's Tail form is directly in front of the opponent who throws a Roundhouse Punch (fig. 8.12). The head is kept slightly low and the arms are initially in Seven Stars (Play the Pi Pa) position. One may find that it is too difficult to get inside a straight jab or strike. However, like most of the Wu style complex patterns, the ideal scenarios remain flexible enough to defend and attack in less-than-ideal situations.

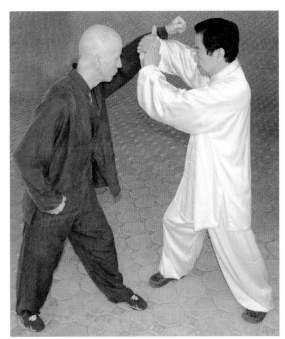

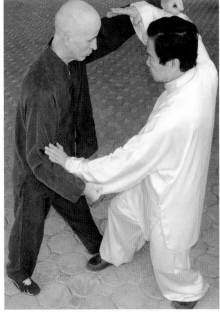

Fig. 8.12. Block and jam using the Bird's Tail form

Developing Discharge Power within the Bird's Tail

It takes time to develop discharge power within the Bird's Tail. The novice learns this complex pattern as three or four separate moves, which can then be combined by more advanced practitioners into a single move. The one move incorporates an outward twist of the waist around the central axis with a slight leaning back of the spine. The tan tien is loaded diagonally from the parry*—in the opposite lower quadrant. From the zenith of the circle, the tan tien rotates back as the practitioner executes a couple of strikes (fig. 8.13). Overall, the move is similar to a tennis serve: the parries are analogous to the wind-up, while power is released in the "serve."

Cross Hands

Cross Hands developed from the Brush Knee form practiced in the Universal Healing Tao Wu Style Short Form. The move combines a double-hands parry with a double strike. The first palm parry guides a punch to a point just beside the adept's head. The second hand makes contact with the dorsum of the hand such that the hands now cross. This cross fits snugly against the opponent's wrist, to the extent that the adept both sticks and locks the opponent's strike. When the stroke reaches its natural zenith, it returns with power from the tan tien to reach the opponent as a double strike; usually it is a Double Punch but could also be a Back Fist with a Punch.

---

*For more information about "loading" the various segments of the tan tien, see *Tan Tien Chi Kung* (Rochester, Vt.: Destiny Books, 2004).

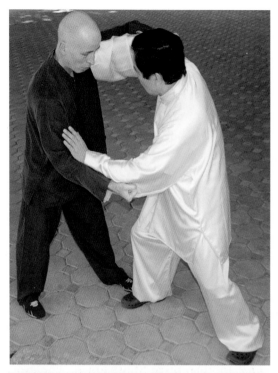

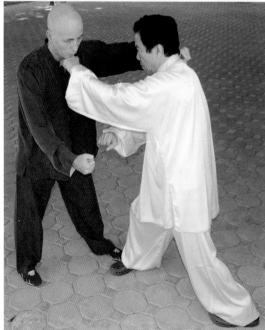

Fig. 8.13. First and second strikes of the Bird's Tail

Deeper Push Hand Principles of Cross Hands

In Tai Chi Boxing, the incoming punches are only marginally deviated so that the opponent stays close and connected and the adept can use the skills of listening and understanding to create an advantage. The Cross Hands parry utilizes principles from Push Hands in that the arms follow and stick. They follow the opponent's force so that it is only minimally deviated from the face. The force is then followed and exaggerated. The adept then uses the Lu force to topple the opponent off balance, or simply delays the opponent's withdrawal to obtain time for a strike.

The Ideal Position for Cross Hands

Cross Hands is best suited to a fully executed punch rather than a feint or jab. The ideal position for executing the move is to be on the blind side of the opponent (fig. 8.14). This position negates any offense from the opponent's other arm or legs. While Cross Hands can be effectively applied to the inside of a punch, this position opens the adept to a higher risk of counterattack from the opponent.

Discharge Power Principles of Cross Hands

Like the Bird's Tail, the complex pattern of Cross Hands begins as several moves that are ultimately combined into one. Beginners are taught four separate moves: block, block, strike, and strike; with the accomplished adept, on the other hand, the block and the strike become indistinguishable, and the sound is more like a machine gun than a series of rifle shots. The movement of jin is similar to that in the Bird's Tail, except that the rotation of the waist is less extreme.

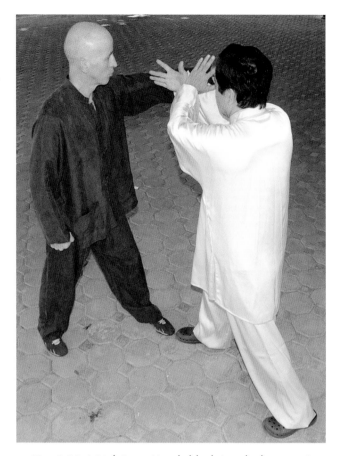

Fig. 8.14. Initial Cross Hands block (in ideal position)

 Willow Tree

Willow Tree is similar to Cross Hands except that the punch or kick is low (see fig. 8.15 on page 210). It is taken from the long form with Parry (Back Fist) and Punch. It is not in the Universal Healing Tao Short Form, however the same principle applies as with Cross Hands in the Brush Knee strike. So it is still possible to learn this application without practicing the long form. It has the spirit of branches of a willow tree flowing in the wind. In this pattern, the arms fold on top of each other and connect, palms down, to the opponent's lower strike or kick. The attack is deviated to the side.

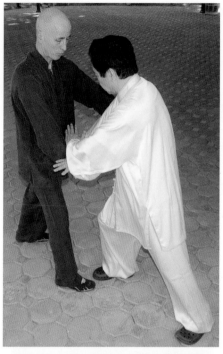

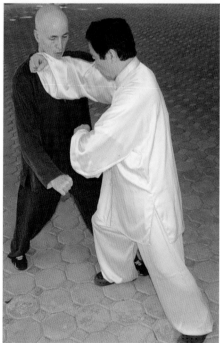

Fig. 8.15. Willow Tree form with follow-up Back Fist

⚙ *The Ideal Position for Willow Tree*

As with Cross Hands, Willow Tree is best used as an entry to the opponent's blind side, thus avoiding a front-on encounter that gives the opponent multiple choices for retaliation. As with most of the boxing techniques, however, Willow Tree is still effective in the front-on position.

⚙ *Push Hands Principles of Willow Tree*

The arms are very relaxed and consequently retain the flexibility to momentarily mold and stick to the opponent's strike. Furthermore, the relaxed arms can cause a painful sting when they are properly employed: it's a paradox that greater relaxation actually brings greater injury to the opponent. The technique finishes with an offensive strike: a Double Punch or a Back Fist and Punch.

⚙ *Discharge Principles of Willow Tree*

The lower cross parry and offensive moves are part of the same release of jin. The tan tien rotates backward with the parries and represents the yin phase of following and listening. The offensive strike is then initiated by the return flick of the tan tien that was set up in the yin phase. Yin feeds yang, and together they become one movement that connects the opponent and the adept to heaven and earth.

Closing the Gate

Closing the Gate is a sequence that is taken from the long form; it is a fusion and modification of the toe kick of the Golden Cock Stands on One Leg and Repulse Monkey. Since this boxing application is not exactly like the form, it does suggest an external influence into the Wu style.

In Closing the Gate, the Cross Hands sequence is combined with an open lower instep (medial arch) kick (fig. 8.16). The Cross Hands can be adapted to suit this technique by placing the open hand further along the opponent's arm—at the elbow. With the waist twisted, the leg closest to the opponent rotates externally and sweeps with force from the tan tien and hip into the opponent's shin or knee. This technique is potent because the kick is below the opponent's field of vision and disguised by movements of the hands above.

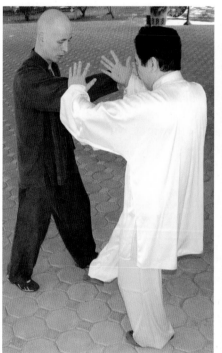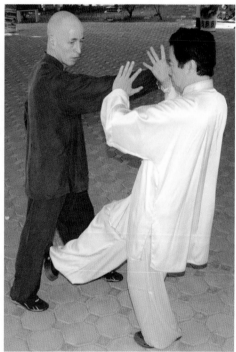

Fig. 8.16. Closing the Gate with instep strike to shin

❂ Ideal Position for Closing the Gate

As with the Cross Hands and Willow Tree techniques, the ideal position for Closing the Gate is on the blind side of the opponent. The same reasoning applies as before.

Discharge Principles of Closing the Gate

Power generated in the leg involves the same principles of discharge as an arm strike. In this sequence, the yin and yang phases are closer together. The yin phase, which lengthens and opens the structure, occurs as the adept follows the opponent's strike to one side, while at the same time cocking and lifting the striking leg to approximately knee height. The cocking of the leg using the empty force creates the right amount of rotation of the hip and foot, creating the structure that will allow the jin to flow. It is consistent with the principle "In the curve seek the straight; store then release."[1] In other words, maximum loading and release of the spring occur when there is appropriate rotation of the foot, ankle, and hip. It also is dependent on a certain degree of flexion of the ankle, knee, and hip. After the tan tien is charged, the power then drives the instep into the opponent's shin or knee.

Single Whip

The Single Whip is part of the Universal Healing Tao Short Form. Its spirit is that of cracking a whip. The waist is considered the handle of the whip; it changes direction and creates a snap in the open palm. In the application of this form, one arm is used to stabilize the opponent's arm while the other strikes. The external manifestations of the form are multiple and can vary considerably from the way they are displayed in the short and long forms.

Ideal Position for Single Whip

The varied shape and application of this form allows for multiple approaches to an opponent. In a front-on position it is not dissimilar to the Bird's Tail opening, in that one arm blocks and traps while the other arm strikes. In the slow form a hook is used; an open palm or a forearm can also replace the hook. In the frontal attack of the Single Whip the striking palm/fist/elbow attacks the other side of the body and can strike the head, neck, chest, abdomen, or limb. In the side or blind position, the trap occurs on the opponent's attacking limb, and the attack strikes a part of the body on the same side.

❂ Discharge Principles of Single Whip

Despite the multiple variations of this move, the simple principle of discharge via the Lieh gate generally applies. The actual anatomical part that ends up striking the opponent is only a minor detail: the foundation is being able to access the jin and use the Lieh force. In the slow form, the yin phase is demonstrated by the sweeping across of the striking palm with rotation of the waist, following and absorbing the opponent's jin into the earth. This move is performed in a relaxed manner that activates the structure through fa song, tucking the sacrum while sinking the abdomen and sternum. The tan tien is then loaded—both by the initial yin rotation and by the jin that naturally rises back from the earth. The fast trap and strike are released in the yang phase using the imagery of the spiral in the lower tan tien.

❂ Push Hands Principles of Single Whip

Push Hands principles apply mostly during the yin phase. For example, if the left hand is the striking palm, then it is the right hand that connects and reads the opponent's energy (ting jin and dong jin). The left hand can then follow an opponent's move or intention and at the required instant—Fa Jin.

INTEGRATION:
BUILDING A BOXING SYSTEM

The building blocks of the boxing forms—the simple and complex moves described above—need to be seeded within the larger arena of physical combat. Integrating the principles from Push Hands into the boxing arena is the next stage in the development of a coherent boxing system. The connections between boxing forms, natural movements of the body, and an unpredictable opponent are all aspects that need developing. To that end, we have created five basic principles.

1. Creating ongoing circles and the central axis
2. Engaging the opponent's strike pattern
3. Following, listening, and understanding
4. Returning to the natural: integrating the body's natural defense reflexes
5. Simplifying and timing the tan tien discharge patterns

Creating Ongoing Circles and the Central Axis

One of the important links required for the fighting system is the creation of circles or orbits. In Push Hands, there is a defined sequence that creates a circle: all techniques are merely tangential departures from this orbit. Our intention is to transplant this principle to the boxing arena.

We must have circles and orbits to connect each of the five complex forms, just as the five basic postures (front, back, right, and left) are connected by a still center. The Seven Stars defense posture can connect to Bird's Tail, Cross Hands, Willow Tree, Single Whip, and Closing the Gate via orbits. In this way the momentum of the arms never ceases—much like electrons around a nucleus.

Each fighter creates another set of orbits. The center is the Tai

Chi pole, which corresponds to the central axis formed by the Central Thrusting Channel in the axial plane (fig. 8.17). In the sagittal plane the center is usually the lower tan tien, though it may sometimes be the heart tan tien.

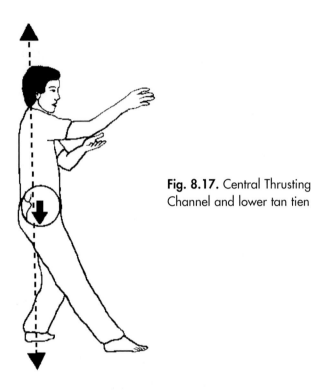

Fig. 8.17. Central Thrusting Channel and lower tan tien

The existence of an opponent also creates two centers, although these two foci gradually merge as the orbits between the practitioners connect (fig. 8.18). A punch begins the circle, which is then observed and connected by the adept. The punch's trajectory is continued like a planet circling the sun, and it is returned to the opponent as a strike. Of course the strikes can vary to include any of the forms or strikes listed above. The circle can range from something that is largely internal in the adept to a clear outward circle. At times, the circle can look like a straight line, though it is actually a circle. Eventually, a new center can be described approximately half way between the opponents.

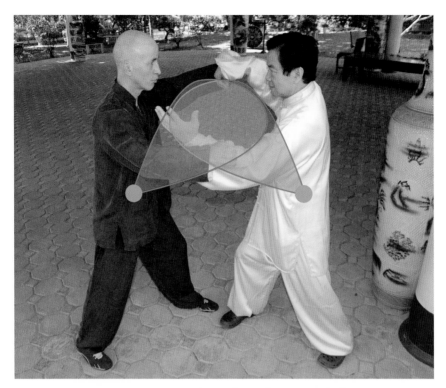

Fig. 8.18. Opponents with circular strike patterns balancing

Engaging the Opponent's Strike Pattern

An important part of developing a boxing system is the establishment of a collection of systematic responses to various classical attacks. These systematic responses are part of what allow the adept to merge with an opponent.

Each of the forms has an ideal position, and each of these positions correlates to a particular quadrant. Forms are applied to front, back, right, left, or center (the five postures), and each of these applications requires a specific response. For example, a Roundhouse Punch to the upper quadrant obligates a Bird's Tail response. A lower strike or kick, on the other hand, invites a Willow Tree sequence to protect the lower quadrant. These relationships mean that the adept has to match various attacks to the various complex forms (see fig. 8.19 on page 218).

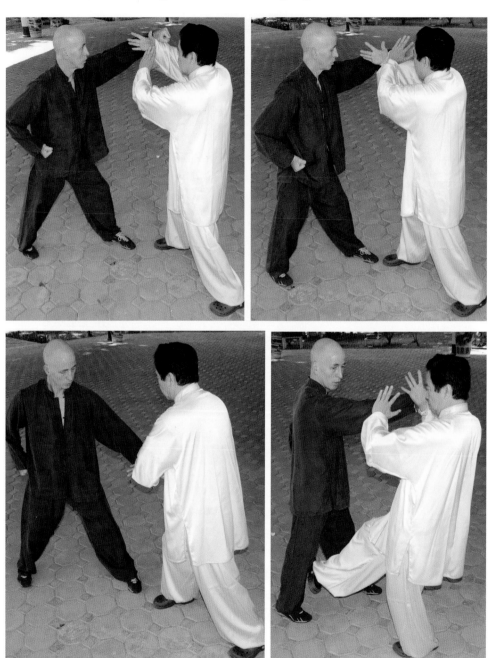

Fig. 8.19. Leading hand setting up Bird's Tail, Cross Hands, Willow Tree, and Instep Kick

A straightforward drill for this level of integration is for a partner to verbally name and thus forewarn the intended form. That is, the opponent will say "Cross Hands" and then deliver a straight punch, which should be countered by the adept's Cross Hands. The opponent can say "Bird's Tail" and then give a Roundhouse Punch, "Willow Tree" to deliver a lower punch, etc.

Once this partner routine has been learned, the opponent can deliver single strikes and blows at defined intervals without prior warning. The intervals can then be reduced or varied to closer mimic the free-sparring situation. Ultimately, the forms will become automatic to a practitioner faced with an attack to a particular quadrant.

IDEAL RESPONSES TO QUADRANT ATTACKS

ATTACK	RESPONSE	IDEAL CIRCUMSTANCES
Upper Quadrants		
Open side Straight Punch	Cross Hands	Not ideal, but can be used
	Single Whip	Punch ideally at lower aspect of upper quadrant
Open side Roundhouse Punch	Bird's Tail	Roundhouse Punch is ideally defended by Bird's Tail
Blind side Straight Punch	Cross Hands	Ideal for head-height punch
	Closing the Gate	Ideal for opponent stepping forward on blind side
Lower Quadrants		
Blind side Kick or low Straight Punch	Willow Tree	Ideal for blind side but not essential
Open side Kick or low Straight Punch	Single Whip	Ideal for strike or kick attacking open side lower quadrants

Following, Listening, and Understanding

The arts of following, listening, and understanding (ting jin, dong jin, and zhang, lian, nian, and sui) are transplanted from Push Hands. Ideally, they rely less on visual input and more on the inner senses: the integrated mind of the adept reaches out and becomes one with the opponent.

Connecting with the opponent through touch, the adept is able to read and predict his next move. This is called dong jin. Theoretically, the kinesthetic sense can be developed to the point where an opponent can be felt from a distance, even when the practitioner's eyes are closed. This ability is touched on in Universal Healing Tao practices of rooting, forming the energy, or connecting to objects of heaven and earth through chi. Most practitioners, however, need to make use of external visual cues in addition to the tactile kinesthetic senses. There are two choices the adept faces when confronting a strike. One involves fear, disconnection, and closing the eyes, while the other involves gentleness, connection, and opening the eyes. Both are natural responses, but the accomplished practitioner obviously chooses the latter.

The adept can choose to follow the force and limb of the opponent with her eyes. The oculomotor reflexes can set up an immediate coordinated response to an opponent's attack that is both natural and faster than any response routed through the intellectual mind. Again, the Wu style lays emphasis on that which is natural and innate. In the long term it is faster, requires no learning, and cannot be forgotten. It is a reflection of the uncarved block, a return from the ten thousand things to the natural way—the Tao.

The eyes will set up the balance center (vestibular system), which then sets up the limbs and spine. (Without the eyes, the body can still maneuver, but with less sensory input—the body and mind are further inclined to error.) The eyes will then arrange the body to a suitable position so that the parry and offensive can begin. The aim of the practitioner is to now merge the startle reflex of the body with the consequences of following with the eyes. The practitioner will notice the creation of something new: a slightly modified, more relaxed, and better-shaped parry. Initial training involves just using a simple single-handed open-palm parry, which the adept can practice until he is successful (fig. 8.20). Then he can begin to add other forms. The opponent can vary the speed and circumstances of her strikes to sharpen the adept's technique. Now, the forms can be initiated and integrated into natural reflexes that reflect both speed and effectiveness.

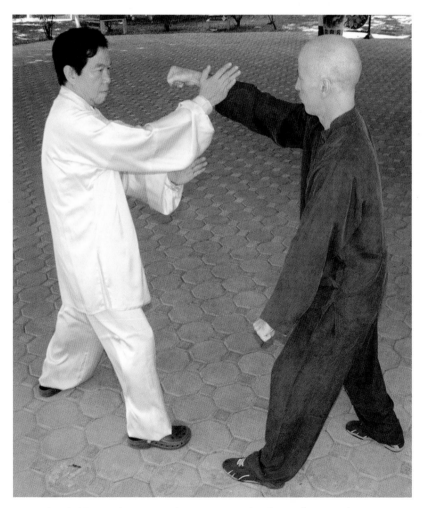

Fig. 8.20. Single open-palm parries to develop reflexes with gaze

Returning to the Natural—
Integrating the Body's Natural Defense Reflexes

Imagine that someone throws an object at you, or moves to hit you from various directions. Then observe how your hands and the body arrange themselves to protect you (fig. 8.21). The next step is to integrate this natural reflex action within the fighting system: parries should be innate rather than artificial movements. The ultimate technique is no technique at all; it is simply natural human movement. We believe this is what the Wu masters Wu Chan-Yu and Wu Jian-Chuan intended.

The student will notice that in self-protection, the hands will take on a Cross Hands shape, with emphasis on the back of the lead hand

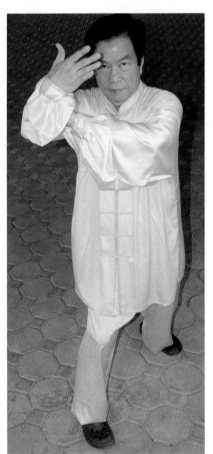

Fig. 8.21. Hands protecting face in a natural reflex response

for self-defense. In an attack, on the other hand—or any attempt to catch or follow an object—the open side of the hand will be used.

Martial engagement is a balance of attack and defense. Furthermore, each defense has an attacking component and each attack a protecting aspect. In parries, the dominant or guiding hand is the open palm capturing (attacking) the opponent's offending strike, while the back of the hand defends. This yin/yang arrangement of the two sides of the hands imitates the body's natural reflex response. It applies to the Bird's Tail, Cross Hands, Willow Tree, Closing the Gate, and Single Whip. In forward offense the hands will also arrange themselves in similar yin/yang patterns.

Simplifying and Timing the Tan Tien Discharge Patterns

The eight gates and the multitude of applications that arise from them can be simplified further. Practiced students will notice that after a while, all the gates merge into a simple flicking of the waist. Grandmaster Wu Gong-Tsao uses the metaphor of refining iron to describe this process. He says, "From raw iron (i.e., iron ore) refined into pipe iron, from pipe iron then refined into pure steel."[2] Refinement is understood as a reversal of the Taoist creation theory and a return to simplicity and the natural.

With this refinement, each tan tien discharge is applied to more and more ideal positions and circumstances in the boxing arena. Initially, we use too much force against an opponent; we use a thousand pounds to beat a thousand pounds. But with refinement of our skills in boxing, we conserve our energy to the point that we can use "four ounces to repel one thousand pounds."[3]

The ability to sustain fighting and mindfulness for prolonged periods is an important aspect of refinement. This ability will often influence outcomes in ring sparring or even street fighting. From an Eastern or Taoist perspective, the ability to relax (fa song) is essential to prolonged fighting. Fa song ensures that minimal energy will be dispersed at each encounter. The adept sweats little and lasts longer than her opponent. While stamina is more a Western concept than an Eastern one, it is worthy of special mention. Stamina can be trained within a Western framework by achieving a calculated heart rate over a sustained period of time.

FINAL AIM

Chang San-Feng believed that boxing was a viable path to ultimate realization of the Tao.[4] We hope that practitioners will recognize that this is the ultimate purpose of Tai Chi Boxing.

In that regard, each of the eight forces represents a separate force in nature; skill develops as each of these forces is recognized and correctly employed. From there comes the ability to interweave each force around a few discharge patterns, an ability to incorporate the theory of substantial and insubstantial, and finally the ability to find a central still point. Competency entails managing this entire skill set.

Ultimately, however, these are not just skills but natural states of being in which the adept remembers how to let go and feel the stillness and peace within, even while the flurry of fighting goes on around him—and even penetrates him at times. Fighting in itself mimics the creation sequence of Taoism: it is the art of becoming nothing. Those that mimic it have found the way; those that forget it are separate. It is not important whether one wins or loses but whether one's actions reflect this profound cosmic principle. Paradoxically, those who embrace this higher principle are the ones who inevitably win.

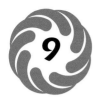

9

Home Practice

Many of the objectives of home practice also apply to other styles of Tai Chi. As discussed in *Tai Chi Fa Jin*, home practice is the cornerstone of self-development and progress in the art. While many improvements are subtle and subjective, they are recognizable to a trained eye, such as a competent Tai Chi judge.

Below is a list of Wu objectives that include both external assessment and internal progress.

- Student displays correct alignment of basic postures and stances that are relaxed and in harmony with internal energies.
- Participant is able to relax and sink energy into the lower tan tien.
- Student's movements are dictated by chi rather than by intellectual intention, and are consequently light, agile, and coordinated.
- Practitioner maintains a posture that allows easier passage of jin. Movements consequently carry power.
- Student displays smooth transition between postures and compliance with the principles of substantial and insubstantial.
- Form encompasses martial meaning.
- Form embodies spirit.
- The student presents well, shows respect, and is well attired.

Progress is measured as the student moves from meditation to standing postures, to the connections between postures in the short form, to simple Push Hands, to a long form, to complex Push Hands, and then to boxing. Wu Gong-Tsao says Tai Chi's "theory of movements and calmness is consistent with sitting Gong . . . it is the moving Gong . . . because it contains the same body of the Tao."[1]

This progression entails mastery not only of chi and jin but also of the body and mind that encompass them. Challenges can be set up to encourage engagement of the art. The adept may choose to up the stakes by entering into interclub or state championships either in Form Display, Push Hands, or boxing tournaments.

The purpose of practicing Tai Chi is not to gain fame or adulation through demonstrations or success in competitions. The purpose of Tai Chi is to discover the Tao. Paradoxically, though, by engaging in competition one can let go of non-Taoist principles such as attachment and fame. Lao Tsu says:

> *Thus we may see*
> *Who cleaves to fame*
> *Rejects what is more great.*[2]

That which is great is the mother of all things, which comes from the Tao. In order to perform well in a competition one needs to not care about winning or losing, or about having a remarkable reputation. Ideally, progress flows from the inside out. As the student opens up his inner energetic worlds, subtle changes occur in his postures and forms. The first step for students is to let go of muscular force and monkey-mind intention. Then awareness of chi gradually improves. Later, the spontaneous appearance of jin occurs, and the laws that govern jin have to be mastered. Finally, the adept experiences the phenomenon of being spirit directed rather than monkey-mind directed. This entails not only being directed like a puppet by the movement of chi but also allowing the emotional and intellectual aspects of the self to be subordinated to the spirit of each form. Ultimately this spirit is one step closer to the source.

The goal of this progression is to get to a point where all manifestations of substantial and insubstantial, closing and opening, and attack and defense are dictated by something beyond. This something beyond is the central theme of the Wu style—the return to the uncarved block that is juxtaposed with the Wu Wei.

From the stillness of the Wu Wei, the spirit of the Wu style is born. While the nature of that spirit is both elusive and ever changing, masters describe it as more feminine, snake-like, and tendon stretching. These descriptions move away from the flamboyance and external power of earlier styles of Tai Chi. The Wu style is something dictated by the chi, jing, shen, and stillness within. Finding that spirit means releasing and having no hold on any aspect of one's being. Letting go is the ultimate way in this inexact spiritual art form.

GOALS OF HOME PRACTICE

Home practice helps us to cultivate the spirit of letting go as we gracefully march through the refinement of static postures, connection between postures, mastering chi and jin, and utilizing the martial spirit.

The Static Postures

The static postures include the five postures of forward (right and left), backward (right and left), and center. They are used in the context of Parallel, Treading, Bow, Horse, Sitting Back, One Leg, and Half Split stances.* Iron Shirt principles can be applied to all of these forms and manifest in the following ways: the neck is long, crown lifted, scapulae rounded, sternum sunk, coccyx and sacrum tucked under, shoulders and elbows down with wrists and fingers loose. The kua is open, and the knees are bent such that a natural height is used.

---

*These are the postures proposed by Tin Chan-Lee in *The Wu Style of Tai Chi Chuan* (Burbank, Calif.: Unique Publications, 1982), 20–26.

Progression through the levels of Iron Shirt entails opening the acupuncture channels and filling the body with chi. As the body fills with chi, the "hollows and projections"[3] disappear. Tension is replaced with softness. The following table describes the achievements that accompany each level of Iron Shirt training.

LEVELS OF IRON SHIRT PRACTICE

LEVEL 1	LEVEL 2	LEVEL 3	LEVEL 4
Student uses muscular effort and the monkey mind or intellect; has no perception of chi.	Beginning to relax and learning to work with gravity. Can use chi in presence of master or on retreat.	Able to open channels with chi in home practice. Able to integrate the three minds into one mind.	Channels open most of the day in everyday life—even in sleep. Three minds merge with spirit.
Multiple blockages in channels.	Hollows and projections disappear on retreat or in presence of master. Student can practice with neck long, shoulders and elbows down, wrists and fingers loose, lumbar back, kua open, knees appropriately flexed. Learning slanted spine postures.	Good Iron Shirt can be experienced alone but still requires warm-up.	Iron Shirt with adept most of the day.
	Reliant on teacher's presence to maintain structure. Tolerates pushing in a couple of postures.	Iron Shirt structure beginning to become second nature. Can tolerate pushes in all classic Wu postures.	Iron Shirt appears naturally in all postures. Can tolerate very strong pushes from multiple persons.
90% yang; postures tense throughout.	70% yang, 30% yin; learning to find power of relaxation (fa song). Tension still appears in postures.	60% yang, 40% yin; tension disappearing, utilizing yang (shaking, intense chi sensations) and yin energies.	50% yang and 50% yin. Balanced energies prevail and almost no tension in the body.

Connections between Postures:
The Immaterial Substances

To the novice observer, the postures would seem to be the foundation of the form, but actually it is the connection between them that builds the common ground and that is paradoxically the unchanging aspect of a Tai Chi form. This is because the connection between postures relies on chi, jin, breath, and spirit, all of which are rooted in stillness and display the cyclical properties of yin and yang. These opposites are called "substantial" and "insubstantial" in Tai Chi and will be discussed in more detail later.

Chi

The flow of chi can be seen in the subtle movements of the form. There is a visible fluid connection between movements in the different joints. When chi opens up the arms, the fingers adjust slightly, and the larger joints move the medium joints, which in turn move the smaller joints. The same happens with the kicks: the foot is adjusted slightly and the leg seems to float up rather than be hoisted up. Li power works the other way and moves the smaller joints first.

Chi keeps connections between disparate parts of the body. For example, in closing movements, when the hand nears the abdomen and pelvis, the abdomen spontaneously sucks in and the kua opens. Every movement becomes a whole-body movement. Wu Yu-Hsiang is a quiet voice in our ear when he says, "Remember, when moving there is no place that doesn't move."[4]

Power or Jin

Even though jin is predominantly an internal phenomenon, it can also be externally observed. It looks like an automatic packing breath that rises smoothly through the body from the earth. Jin inflates and packs the body while at the same time screwing and rotating it in various ways to allow maximum strength and discharge power. Unlike the artificial packing that novices practice in Iron Shirt training, the movement of jin is a spontaneous wavelike phenomenon.

As jin rises from the earth, the legs externally rotate at the hips, the coccyx tucks underneath, the tan tien inflates circumferentially, the spine moves back from bottom to top, the scapulae round, the shoulder externally rotates, and the elbows drop. This jin passes like a wave without obstruction from the feet to the fingertips. The body appears to rise and fall with this movement of power.

Shen

Shen is the final immaterial substance to enter each posture or form. Because the spirit can be gently guided through the crown, it's important to open the crown and keep "suspending the head-top."[5] The will of the practitioner must let go. All details that have been learned must now be forgotten. This could include: foot placement, knee positioning, hip rotation, use of the waist, and placement of consciousness. This all must be forgotten now and replaced with trust in spirit.

This final refinement is a recurring concept in the martial arts. Many grading systems (belts) progress from white to yellow, then to green, orange, and finally black. Within the black belt there are grades of black or dans. Bruce Lee believed that if we followed the principle of letting go and being spontaneous, then the accomplished martial artist would gain a white belt at the highest level.*

The skills, mind training, stances, and applications must all be forgotten. The student returns whence he came: to a state of no expectations or limitations—like a beginner who fights in a natural way, albeit poorly. For a while, the journey through the grades probably makes the adept a worse fighter or clumsier one, but as the skills and knowledge are slowly integrated he advances. The final stage is about letting go and becoming spontaneous. It is similar to the beginning and a return to the natural.

It is important to note, however, that being spontaneous and

---

*Though this may seem paradoxical, what he means is that at the highest level you return to where you started from—spontaneity!

natural has further dimensions. Letting go is ultimately about letting spirit enter you. This is a way of acknowledging the lack of separation between life forms. The spirits of animals (tiger, crane, and so on), work (Fair Lady Works the Shuttle), and the elements (Wave Hands like Clouds, Needle at the Sea Bottom) are not separate from us; in the Taoist theory spirit animates all beings.

The spirit descends through the crown or up from the earth and resides in the organs (fig. 9.1). The chief spirit is the Shen, which resides in the heart. The other spirits are Beibei (spleen), Yanyan (lungs), Fu Fu (kidneys), and Jianjian (liver).[6]

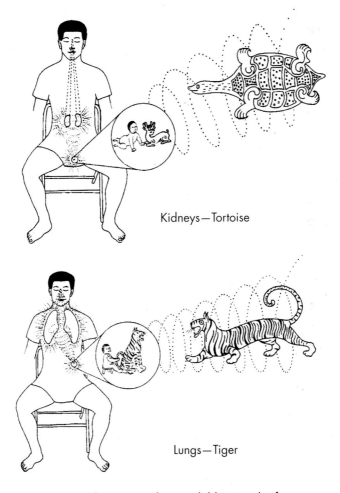

Kidneys—Tortoise

Lungs—Tiger

Fig. 9.1. Animal spirits (and inner children) in the five organs

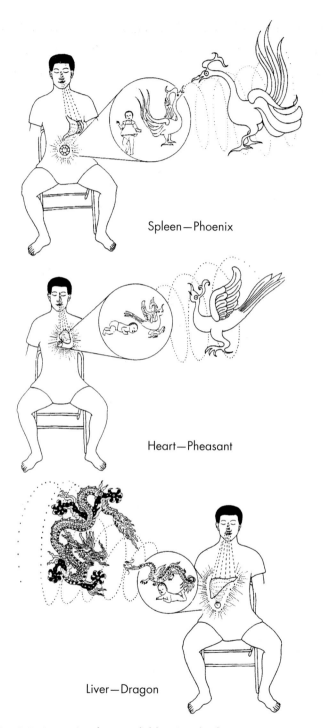

Spleen—Phoenix

Heart—Pheasant

Liver—Dragon

Fig. 9.1. Spirits (and inner children) in the five organs, continued

In the Fusion meditations, the student reconnects to the standard totem animals associated with the organs—the heart's red pheasant, the spleen's phoenix, the white tiger of the lungs, the tortoise or deer of the kidneys, and the green dragon of the liver (fig. 9.2).

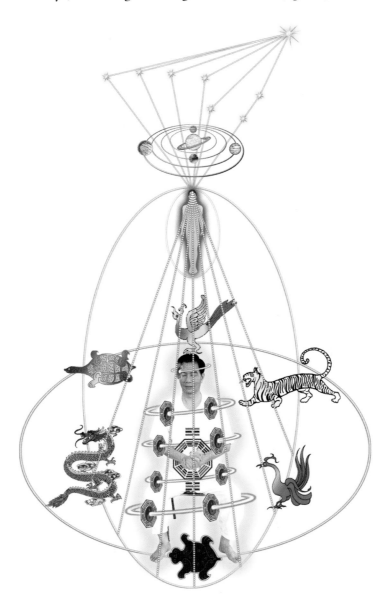

Fig. 9.2. The Fusion meditations connect the student with the totem animal for each organ.

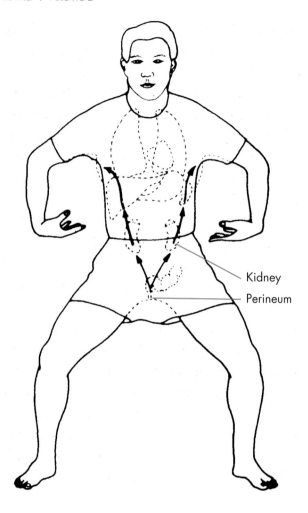

Kidney

Perineum

Fig. 9.3. Golden Phoenix posture

In Iron Shirt training, the student is exposed to the Golden Turtle, Golden Phoenix (fig. 9.3), and the Buffalo.

Animal spirits are also invoked in the Greater Kan and Li course, when students extend their awareness deep into the center of the earth to access animal spirits. Initially, students just visualize the spirits, but they must be embodied in order to perfect the forms. This is the way of the shaman, who channels animal spirits in order to access powers and knowledge of the divine.

The external manifestation of spirit can be seen in the eyes of the practitioner and in the nature of a movement. Spirit defines the character of a movement series into something recognizable. For example, a sequence of moves of various joints could be fairly mechanical and dry, yet with spirit this same sequence can take on the energy of a crane, roc bird, or a whip. While chi can move the joints and body in a fluid manner, and jin can expand the body and make it strong, it is the spirit that gives the body character. Spirit returns the body to nature via the wonderment of the human imagination.

In Taoist esoteric arts, the allocation of particular spirits to particular forms follows stereotypes and established culture. For the Western student exploring these arts, it is not necessary to keep to this standard repertoire. Be like a child and play. Join a drama group and discover the realm of spirit!

The best gauge of success in channeling an animal spirit is the adept's own individual perception. One feels light, out of control, animated, and coordinated beyond everyday awareness. One becomes something else! To the spectator, the performer will appear to have a presence, which is often something beyond words. This X factor will be seen in the subtle features of the eyes, hands, coordination, and whole-body movement. The attention of the spectator will be captured, and the link to the divine acknowledged.

Martial Meaning

Martial meaning is another layer of information that needs to be explored first on its own, then integrated with the mind, chi, jin, breath, and spirit. Martial meaning is learned from classroom teachings and educational resources like books and videos. Applications are taught to the intellectual mind and are then learned in a staged and fragmented way with partner work and home practice. Eventually, the body internalizes the applications and can institute a defense without thought. The integrated mind allows the whole body to connect to an inner image. This is a useful way to practice the slow form—letting the imagination work with the body to execute the form in various martial scenarios. Ultimately, applications become a spontaneous event involving the whole body and imagination. An outside observer assessing your form will see each posture filled with appropriate martial intention. The martial intention attracts the right spirit and relevant use of chi and jin.

Breath

Breath mirrors the interplay of yin and yang that heralds the stillness of the supreme ultimate. However, this kind of breathing doesn't happen right away; in the novice, the breath is all over the place. The practitioner is tense and the center of gravity is high. Respirations are rapid and involve expansion and contraction of the chest only. The use of muscular force results in the holding of the breath, which must catch up sooner or later with a period of panting.

With time and the incorporation of some principles of fa song, the breath starts to descend to the abdomen. The practitioner may have enough control to inhale with closing movements and exhale with outward movements. The sound of the breath remains audible to the outside observer and indicates to the competent judge where the student is at.

Later, with further relaxation, the breath becomes silent. It coordinates with movement and the phenomenon of whole-body breathing appears (fig. 9.4). Breath is now interlaced with the Iron Shirt structure. Now, when the whole body breathes, every muscle from the pinkie toe to the top of the scalp is involved. Breath links to the movement of chi, and the cycle of chi is in turn linked with movement. Inhalation is linked with closing moves (retreat), while exhalation is associated with opening moves (attack). Closing moves activate the empty force breath while opening moves are associated with the packing breath and jin. While the breath is normally cyclical, there may be times when it completely disappears or explodes with the release of Discharge Power.

To the outside observer, the adept student is not overtly breathing. The form becomes a cyclical interplay of yin and yang as the substantial and insubstantial. Finally, breath is spontaneous and totally forgotten.

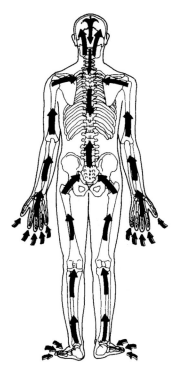

Fig. 9.4. Whole-body breathing

The following table summarizes the various dimensions that need to be developed and integrated into home practice.

DIMENSIONS OF HOME PRACTICE

	LEVEL 1	LEVEL 2	LEVEL 3	LEVEL 4
MIND	Uses muscular effort, uses the monkey mind or intellect.	Learning to sink awareness into the lower tan tien.	Integrating and developing the three minds. Mind moves the chi, which moves the limbs. Mind and jin beginning to coordinate.	Mind integrated with the dimensions of spirit, chi, and jin. Mind is without thought and takes on the direction of spirit, which moves the chi and jin.

	LEVEL 1	LEVEL 2	LEVEL 3	LEVEL 4
BODY (IRON SHIRT STRUCTURE)	Body disconnected. Multiple blockages in forms and between postures. Forces are not aligned. Easily pushed over and can't take a punch to any part of the body without pain.	"Hollows and projections" beginning to disappear in postures. On occasions, structure is still excessively forward or backward. Can take a strike to lower abdomen only.	Most forms show good Iron Shirt structure. Good connections between forms. Jin passes from the legs through the waist, spinal column, and then to the hands. Can take pushes in most postures. Iron Shirt spreading to back and chest; can take blows there.	Ideal structure in all forms, with constant and steady center and upright posture. Can take pushes in all postures from all directions. Able to take blows to all parts of the body.
CHI	Multiple breaks in form. Li power means small joints lead the large joints. No connection between different parts of the body. No awareness of chi!	Segments of connection and continuity of forms. Muscles are more relaxed and movements naturally slow. Senses chi in the hands and isolated segments of the body.	Grace and chi engaged in some forms with ongoing continuity. Chi is listened to and followed, and moves the larger joints first. Different parts of the body seem to be connected. Connections between chi and jin.	Chi is directed by the spirit which engages the jin. Body moves with grace and softness at an ideal tempo.
BREATH	Breath is labored and loud.	Breath is becoming connected to the form, with yin movements on inhalation and closing movements on exhalation.	Whole-body breathing: breath almost disappears to an observer.	Breath is spontaneous yet quiet and easy. Breath is linked with chi, jin, and spirit of each form. In closing forms the breath ceases and empty force activates. In opening forms, the breath packs the body naturally. In phase 8 of Fa Jin the breath is released from the whole body in a climaxlike discharge.

	LEVEL 1	LEVEL 2	LEVEL 3	LEVEL 4
MARTIAL MEANING	Applications not understood or portrayed.	Some intellectual understanding of meaning and applications.	Meaning becomes apparent through placement of head, arms, waist, and legs. Able to use imagination to enact forms in various martial scenarios.	Higher awareness creates a deep (body and mind) understanding of martial applications for each form. Each part of the adept's form is embellished with a rich and variant martial meaning.
JIN	Li power only.		Able to consciously pack the body in segments. Glimpses of spontaneous packing or inflation of the body with jin. No connection between chi and jin yet.	Awareness of Xu Jin (gathering power in closing movements) and Fa Jin in occasional forms and gates. Occasional connections between chi and jin. Still has blockages where jin cannot pass through.
SPIRIT	Stuck in monkey mind; no access to spiritual dimension.	Learning to mimic animals, the elements, and actions of people.	Episodic use of a limited range of spirits to coordinate forms.	Rooted in stillness, able to access to a large range of spirits to execute attacking or defensive moves.

Manifesting the Principles of the Substantial and Insubstantial

A key indicator of progression in Tai Chi is the student's ability to manifest the principles of substantial and insubstantial. The judge or teacher may get an idea of the internal progress through intuition, but she essentially relies on external signs. Many of these external signs have been discussed in this text, however, they have not been collated from a purely substantial and insubstantial viewpoint.

These external signs can be summarized in table form and include:

SUBSTANTIAL AND INSUBSTANTIAL (EXTERNAL SIGNS)

QUALITY	INSUBSTANTIAL/YIN	SUBSTANTIAL/YANG
	Closing	Opening
Stages of discharge	4 yin phases (Xu Jin)	4 yang phases (Fa Jin)
	Absorption	Discharge
Martial quality	Retreat	Advance
	Parry	Attack
	Void	Embodied
Spirit	Calm	Vital
	Eyes relaxed	Eyes wide
	Eyes inward	Eyes to imaginary opponent
Awareness	Inward	Outward
Chi in the body	Empty	Full
Posture	Rooted	Lifting
Breath	Inward	Outward
Overall movement	Stillness	Activity
	Slow	Fast

These external signs need to be acknowledged but not rigidly exercised. They can provide feedback to the student about his inner progress, but they are not the essence of Tai Chi: one could never consciously put all the disparate pieces together. Sometimes, however, a teacher can chisel away at some of these external qualities and take the student back to the essence. This is especially so with the cultivation of yin. We often encourage students to be slow, calm, and empty. We ask them to connect to the earth, relax the eyes, and absorb. These yin qualities will help them discover the inner essence of Tai Chi.

The yin qualities are not endpoints in themselves, however. Slowness, for example, is a yin quality, but it is not the purpose of doing the Tai Chi form. If slowness were the purpose, then taking one hour to do a long form would be a logical goal. The purpose of doing the form slowly is to awaken other aspects of being—the internal senses and, later, the awareness of chi and jin. Slowness may help the practitioner discover chi and jin, but it is not a goal in itself.

The essence of Tai Chi is stillness and calmness, which are cultivated through standing and sitting meditation. From stillness the chi is born. Chi obeys the cyclical laws of yin and yang. To emphasize this point, Wu Gong-Tsao says, "Taijiquan follows the theory of the Taiji's movements and calmness as the methods, uses the marvellous variations of the insubstantial and substantial as the applications."[7]

The Cycles of Chi and Jin

The cycles of chi and jin movement have been discussed throughout this text, but for a moment let us emphasize the cyclical nature of this movement. As we exhale, the body becomes yang and is inflated with jin. Movements open and ultimately jin disperses. From this dispersed state, the senses gather chi while the body inhales and closes; the chi then retreats to the tan tien and the earth. The body becomes still. From this stillness the cycle begins again.

Spirit is also involved in this cycle. It enters the body during the stillness and can exit upon discharge of jin or stay in the body if the subsequent moves are suited to it. For example, multiple moves in the Bird's Tail may incorporate the same spirit.

PUSH HANDS

Push Hands in the Wu style is very similar to the Yang style. The subtle differences are reflected in the basic postures, which tend to be less square while allowing a greater slant to the spine. The sequences of Push Hands can be found in *Tai Chi Fa Jin** and will not be repeated here. However, it is worthwhile to summarize the markers of progress for home practice.

---

*Mantak Chi and Andrew Jan, *Tai Chi Fa Jin* (Rochester, Vt.: Destiny Books, 2012).

External Markers

The student first learns single-handed Push Hands and then learns two-handed practice. Within the routine, the student learns how to change directions, have strength in the five postures, and grasp the intentions of the eight gates. Once this is familiar, the adept forgets about the routine and concentrates on the subtleties of following and interpreting. Once the eight gates have been learned by the intellectual mind, the rest of the body must memorize them.

Initially, the student is awkward: the monkey mind is not capable of mastering the art of Push Hands. The intellect cannot interpret and understand an opponent's movement; only the integrated three minds can do this. The novice's structure is poor and he has trouble sitting back (fig. 9.5). When the kua and kidneys are weak then the student will tend to bob up and down, moving forward and backward. He will stoop forward and lean too far back. Eventually, however, the student can apply principles of good structure to a moving

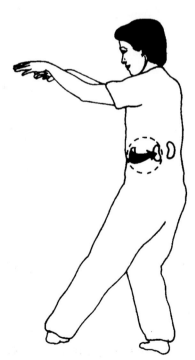

Fig. 9.5. Sitting back with full-kidney posture

situation. In Push Hands, you win if you maintain your structure and you lose if you do not.

Initially, internal power is incomprehensible. With time, practice, and understanding, however, the student learns how to correctly release power from the earth through the body. Likewise, learning to read an opponent's structure through touch (following, listening, and understanding jin) occurs with time and devotion (fig. 9.6). It is

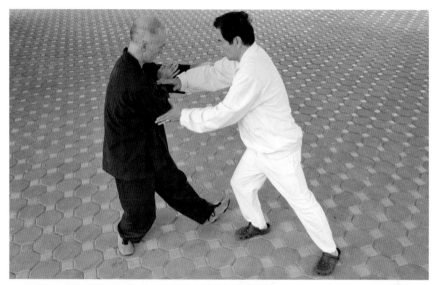

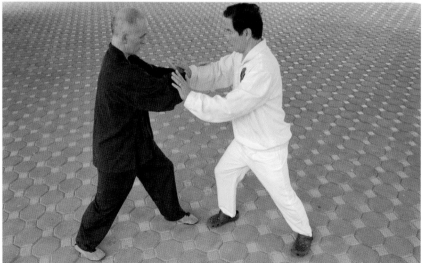

Fig. 9.6. Push Hands: practicing following, listening, and understanding

a giant leap forward when the adept realizes the power of relaxation and becomes able to attune himself to his opponent and the forces around him.

It is important that the student Push Hands with multiple opponents of varying skill levels. The variation requires the student to remain spontaneous and to not premeditate an attack or defense. Each opponent will have different skills and weaknesses, which will strengthen the Push Hands armory of the adept.

Subjective Internal Markers

After spending a couple of years learning the routines——the skills of listening, understanding, and the use of the eight gates of discharge——Push Hands becomes like a meditation in itself. The multiple avenues of sensory input are reduced by the integrated three minds to a primordial perception. The adept's mind merges with the opponent's body and interprets its structure for any faults. The adept's body spontaneously reacts with an exaggeration of the defects to culminate in successful discharge.

PUSH HANDS LEVELS

LEVEL 1	LEVEL 2	LEVEL 3	LEVEL 4
Learning the routine	Relaxing into the routine	Using opponent's movements as guide	Using spirit to guide movements
Uses the monkey mind with predetermined ideas	More relaxed but still keeping a move in mind	Following, interpreting, and listening	Truly spontaneous, appears to read an opponent even before he moves; mind of adept merges with opponent's mind
Broken structure: difficulty sitting back and center moves up and down	Four faults of butting, deficiency, breaking, and stiffness	Faults disappear, good structure in the five steps	Soft and alive in all positions

LEVEL 1	LEVEL 2	LEVEL 3	LEVEL 4
Uses muscles and Li power; power is disconnected from opponent	Power still fragmented; breakages in link between earth, legs, waist, spine, and arms	Power is aligned and connected to opponent's force	Transmits power from the earth, borrows power from the opponent, releases power when only "four ounces" are required
Learning eight gates	Learning eight gates, becoming familiar with a few	Familiar with all eight gates	Eight gates include Fa Jin

BOXING

The student progresses through boxing in much the same way as he or she does through the short or long form.

Level 1

To begin with, basic martial strikes are taken out of the slow form and practiced—with mitts and gloves—in real time with real force. At the same time, the student continues to work on her Iron Shirt, slow form, Push Hands, and of course chi and jin training.

Level 2

In level 2, the student learns to put complex patterns together. What was initially learned by the intellectual mind is repeated numerous times until the body has a memory of the pattern. With time, the sequence melts into one move. With more time and practice, the student learns to let chi and jin enter each form. Now, when the student practices with a partner, the contacts between them can sting.

Level 3

In level 3, the student begins to integrate in all aspects of the training. In Iron Shirt practice, the student begins to find the Central Thrusting Channel and can easily rotate around it. In Push Hands, the practitioner can effectively read an opponent through touch.

In Southern Wu style fighting, close contact is encouraged. This enables the adept to predict the opponent's next move as well as to sense when the opponent is off balance. In boxing, the student learns how to follow with his eyes. He knows the ideal scenario for each pattern so that each form fits together in the tapestry of free fighting.

Level 4

In level 4, the adept has reached mature stages of the art, and all of her skills fuse into natural and spontaneous actions. There are no methods or fixed rules anymore. What was learned is now forgotten. The adept can read opponents through the subtle realms of energy and spirit. Each attack is laden with jin and spirit but more than that—the opponent and the adept have become one.

SUMMARY OF BOXING LEVELS

LEVEL 1	LEVEL 2	LEVEL 3	LEVEL 4
Basic Strikes	Complex Forms	Integration	Mastery
Palm Strike	Bird's Tail	Ongoing circles and central axle	Spontaneity
Punching	Cross Hands	Following opponent's strikes with the eyes	Reads opponent using following, listening, and understanding
Back Fist (or Back Fist and Punch)	Willow Tree	Listening and understanding through physical contact	Multitude of techniques from long form include Iron Shirt for defense

LEVEL 1	LEVEL 2	LEVEL 3	LEVEL 4
Variant punches: Roundhouse, Uppercut	Close the Gate	Appropriate forms for each attack	Multitude of attacks from long form
Silk-reeling parries	Single Whip	Appropriate timing: 4 ounces topples a thousand pounds	Operates at level of chi, jin, and spirit

HARMONIZING WITH NATURAL CYCLES

Home practice eventually becomes the focus of the day and shines over whatever portion of the day is seemingly not Tao practice. This includes our sleeping, working, eating, and socializing. When we juxtapose our daily practice upon the natural cycles of the day, we somehow merge with cycles of the sun, moon, and planets—even with our universe's cycle of expansion (post Big Bang) and contraction (Big Crunch). By participating in natural cycles we participate in the dance of the Tao, which in turn enhances our Tai Chi and ancillary Taoist practices.

Daily Cycles

Each hour of the day has a certain quality of energy that reflects the interplay and harmony of the five elements. Each element connects to an internal organ, particular emotions, our thinking life, and bodily functions. Tap into these connections and notice maximum benefit; go against them and consequently become frustrated, ineffectual, and blocked. Man is not separate from the universal forces and should not try to be. Cultivating balance and harmony requires following, listening, and understanding nature's cycles. These three words sound familiar; they are the same three words we use to describe the art of Push Hands. Further descriptions cultivate stillness and yin. Our society with its yang approach of doing negates tapping into this cosmic power. By being soft and still, one may find that the yang side of our lives is more explosive and powerful.

The following table provides a summary of the chi cycle in relation to an ideal daily life. However, please note that each individual is blessed with a particular blend of organ energies and while this provides a useful guide, one size does not fit all!

DAILY CYCLES OF THE ORGANS

TIME	ORGAN	RECOMMENDED ACTIVITIES	ORGAN FUNCTIONS
5–7 a.m.	**LARGE INTESTINE**	Getting ready for the day. Heavenly and earthly chi is pouring into the body like a rapidly flowing river. Activities should assist the embodiment of dreams. This time is a bridge between the spirit world and earthly worlds. Begin with light meditation, chi weight lifting, Empty Force Breath, warm-ups, Tai Chi, and Chi Kung. Finish with meditation.	
7–9 a.m.	**STOMACH**	The time that the energetic dimension meets the material world of tastes, nourishment, warmth, and splendor! Cooked breakfast is best—the main meal of the day.	The earth element governs the digestion and absorption of chi. It also holds the center, providing peace and nourishment.
9–11 a.m.	**SPLEEN**	Action time: hard work, earthly problem-solving time, meetings with others, and healing of others. Absorption of chi continues with reading and writing—including study of the classics. Fulfillment of your grounded earthly mission.	

TIME	ORGAN	RECOMMENDED ACTIVITIES	ORGAN FUNCTIONS
11 a.m.– 1 p.m.	**HEART**	Creativity and hard work continue. Follow your heart and exercise the spirit that lives in your heart. Here you will find true internal power.	Creativity: heart yin begets insight while heart yang expresses it. Spirit resides in the heart during the day (and in the liver at night).
1–3 p.m.	**SMALL INTESTINE**	Time for lunch and the start of the yin phase. Take the opportunity to switch off with a power nap or brief meditation.	The small intestine purifies the creativity of the heart.
3–5 p.m.	**BLADDER**	Time for activities that are more mundane and require little mind power. Exercise in the afternoon may be a waste of time.	
5–7 p.m.	**KIDNEY**	Time to detoxify from work and nurture the kidneys. This is good time to gather some rejuvenation, including sexual practices. Kidney yin lubricates the jin. Kidney chi helps to receive air chi (*zhong chi*) and combine it with stomach digestion chi (*ku chi*) and Original Chi (*yuan chi*).	The combination of kidney yang and kidney chi forms willpower.[8] Kidney power gives us strength in the lower back, connects the adept to the earth, and also helps in knowing when to retreat.
7–9 p.m.	**PERICARDIUM**	Home time: time to protect the heart. Be with family, friends, and Taoist buddies over a light evening meal. Best to go to bed slightly hungry. Do winding down exercises—ideally on the floor—including Tao Yin and the Six Healing Sounds.	Pericardium yin protects the spirit by closing the heart. The pericardium helps to find the right teacher and colleagues for safe creative expression.
9–11 p.m.	**TRIPLE WARMER**	Time to fall asleep. The triple warmer disperses chi and moves you into new dimensions where you can discover your true identity.	The triple warmer distributes energy evenly between the three cavities of the body, creating balance and warmth. It prevents extremes of thoughts and behavior.

TIME	ORGAN	RECOMMENDED ACTIVITIES	ORGAN FUNCTIONS
11 p.m. –1 a.m.	**GALLBLADDER**	Sleep time	
1–3 a.m.	**LIVER**	Restoration time: you should be in a total yin state, fast asleep. This is when the ethereal soul (*hun*) ventures off to the spirit world to converse with Immortals and past masters. "This is the time when the unconscious is supreme."[9] The Hun passes its information to the corporeal soul (*po*).	Movement energy: liver yang is action. Liver yin allows us to retreat and wait. The liver provides "the wisdom to know when to move and when to be still."[10] It governs the eyes, tendons, ligaments, and storage of blood.
3–5 a.m.	**LUNGS**	This is the grand time: the corporeal soul (po) brings the information and inspiration from the spirit world—and the magic of the world of dreams—back into the body.	Letting go (yang) and reattachment (yin).

Weekly Cycles

Each week manifests another set of cycles. This knowledge is embedded in the names of our days, though sometimes these associations are clearer in the French or Spanish names (shown in parentheses). Monday (lundi, lunes) is Moon day, Tuesday (mardi, martes) is Mars day, Wednesday (mecredi, miércoles) is Mercury day, Thursday (jeudi, jueves) is Jupiter day, Friday (vendredi, viernes) is Venus day, Saturday is Saturn day, and Sunday is Sun day (fig. 9.7). It is helpful to arrange your week so that your activities fit in with these planetary rulers: Monday is ruled by the moon and is consequently emotional and changeable; give space for these changes and keep your bookings flexible. Tuesday is ruled by Mars and is therefore a great day for fighting, action, and making changes. Try to practice your boxing and Push Hands with colleagues on this day; it's also a great day to book those appointments where conflict is necessary. Wednesday is a time for thinking, writing, and studying the classics of Tai Chi

and Taoism. Thursday is associated with the biggest planet—
Jupiter—and hence is time for solving some of the biggest philo-
sophical questions within the Tao. Friday is dominated by Venus and
is to be reserved for love. Saturday belongs to Saturn and is therefore a time for organizing (home affairs and maintenance). Sunday
belongs to the center and should be a day of stillness and rest.

WESTERN DAY/PLANET CORRESPONDENCES

DAY	RELATED PLANET
Sunday	Sun
Monday	Moon
Tuesday	Mars
Wednesday	Mercury
Thursday	Jupiter
Friday	Venus
Saturday	Saturn

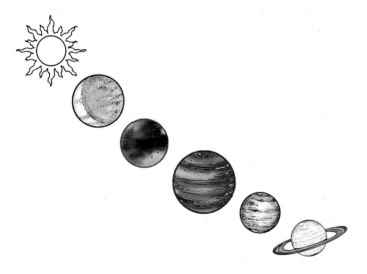

Fig. 9.7. The days of the week and their corresponding planets

The days and their planetary associations are similar in Chinese astrology, but the symbolism is different. Both the five elements and the fundamental aspects of yin and yang influence the days. Some authors also suggest that the days are influenced by the Chinese zodiac animals (according to the twelve-year-cycle of Jupiter).* In the Chinese systems—as in the Western ones—each day will bear a spirit or principle that seekers should align with for maximum prosperity. It is important to remember, however, that each person has a unique blend of planetary endowments and will be affected by specific energies in different ways.

CHINESE DAY/PLANET CORRESPONDENCES

DAY	PLANET	ELEMENT/PRINCIPLE	ANIMAL
Monday	Moon day	Yin/feminine	Goat
Tuesday	Mars day	Fire	Dragon
Wednesday	Mercury day	Water	Horse
Thursday	Jupiter day	Wood	Pig and rat
Friday	Venus day	Metal	Snake, dog, and rabbit
Saturday	Saturn day	Earth	Tiger, ox, and rooster
Sunday	Sun day	Yang/masculine	Monkey

Seasonal Cycles

Within the year there are the seasons, which are overtly linked to the five-element cycle (fig. 9.8). Spring is for expansion and new projects. Winter is a time for quiet inner work and self-reflection. Autumn is a time for culling activities and material belongings, while

---

*See: www.chineseastrologer.org; viewed January 2011.

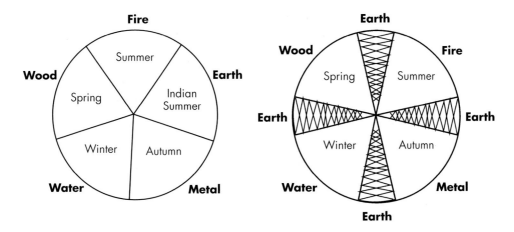

Fig. 9.8. Earth Seasons

summer is a time for shining. Indian summer is the center of the year around which all else revolves.*

The Eight Pillars of Health

More important than any astrological correspondences, however, is to be sensitive to your own thoughts, feelings, and past experiences and to use this inner knowledge to maximize chi and health in your body. Good health is a fundamental part of the Chinese internal arts, as progress cannot be made if there is sickness in the body or other significant problems. The eight major pillars of health are: Tai Chi (Chi Kung), good sleep and rest, good food and digestion, good water, balanced emotions, loving sexuality/relationship, good vocation, and good spiritual connections (see fig. 9.9 on page 254).

There are many ways of understanding these pillars and many systems that include additional pillars or different ones. Some authors include detoxification and herbal/mineral supplements as extra pillars,[11] whereas we would suggest that these are part of the

---

*For more detailed information about Chinese astrology, see Mantak Chia and Dirk Oellibrandt, *Taoist Astral Healing* (Rochester, Vt.: Destiny Books, 2004).

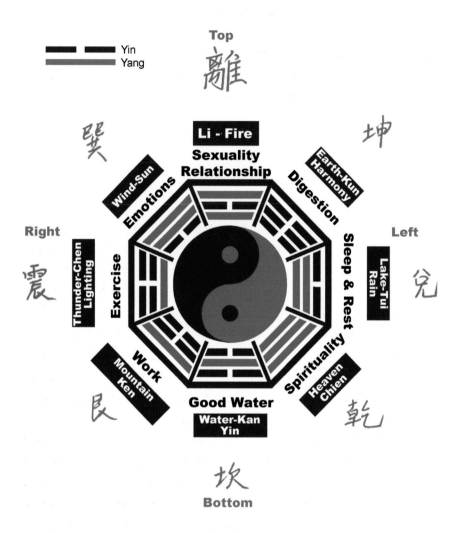

Fig. 9.9. The pakua and the eight pillars of health

Chi Kung and good food/digestion categories. Ayurveda highlights three to five pillars, which include food, sex, sleep/rest, work, exercise, and relationship. From a Taoist perspective, housing could also be in the mix, as a healthy house also influences health significantly. Sexuality could also be regarded as the force that combines or fuses the eight components rather than a pillar on its own. Nevertheless, breaking down the major components of health into sectors is a useful exercise.

In order to maintain the benefits Chi Kung and Tai Chi (and acupuncture, for those receiving treatments) one needs the replenishing aspect of the other pillars and in particular food and/or herbs to fix them.

THE TAO OF DIGESTION

The Chinese or Taoist approach to nutrition incorporates many dimensions. At a simple mechanical level, the body is understood to require certain basic components to fuel cellular growth and repair. At a more refined level, eating and digestion can be experienced as an artistic celebration of the material plane. In any case, nutritional needs are different for students participating in everyday society than they are for those advanced practitioners who have withdrawn from everyday life and are totally devoted to Tao practice. While there are specific dietary recommendations for the latter group, they are beyond the scope of this text, which is geared toward students who choose to live in society as healthfully as possible.

The simple mechanical model lies at the bottom of the pyramid of refinement but is nevertheless of vital importance. It is not too dissimilar from the Western framework that breaks foods down into carbohydrates, proteins (amino acids), fiber, fatty acids, nucleic acids, essential vitamins, and minerals. Chinese medicine regards the essential components of food as sources of various types of chi. These types of chi supply the five major organs with yin and yang chi, create an ideal internal temperature, and help to direct and move chi within the body.

Some examples of foods that include various types of chi are included in the following table. Classification is problematic at times, and variation among different texts is considerable.*

---

*For a detailed and excellent thorough analysis, the authors recommend Paul Pitchford's text *Healing with Whole Foods: Oriental Traditions and Modern Nutrition* (Berkeley, Calif.: North Atlantic Books, 1993).

FOOD CHI SUPPORTS THE ORGANS

ORGAN	YIN FOODS	YANG FOODS	TASTE	COLOR
Heart	Whole grain rice, mushrooms, chamomile, jujube seeds	Red Meats	Bitter	Red
Spleen	Rice congee, oats (cooked)	Carbohydrate-rich vegetables	Sweet	Yellow
Lungs	Dairy products (small amounts), sweet rice, pear, apple	Onion, peppers	Pungent	White
Kidneys	Oysters, shellfish, kidney beans, bone marrow soup, seaweeds	Kidney offal, royal jelly	Salty	Black
Liver	Tofu, berries, seaweed, rhubarb root	Ginger, horseradish	Sour	Green

Heating and Cooling

Food is also classified according to its effects on the body after digestion. For example, foods that make you sweat while eating paradoxically cool the body for hours later. Ice cream may seem initially cooling on a hot day, but it is actually warming over the long term because the body creates exothermic heat in an attempt to digest the fat. In other words, don't be persuaded by the immediate sensations or rewards of any particular food; explore the responses of your body for hours after you've eaten. Dietary choice should be an attempt to balance the internal milieu well beyond the meal.

Depending on your constitution and the external weather patterns, you may choose foods that are heating, neutral, or cooling. Foods that produce heat are included in the yang section of the above table and include: chili, garlic, onion, curries, pepper, red meat, and brown rice. Drying, frying, grilling, and baking foods increases their heating potency. Foods that come from beneath the earth are great for winter warming—think of potatoes, carrots, turnips, and other roots and tubers.

Cooling foods include fruit, steamed foods, salads, green vegetables, and white meats. Preparation modes that do not add heat include steaming, soups, and porridge. Raw foods can be cooling or heating: if the raw food is difficult to digest then it can produce some heat.

The Five Flavors

Foods are classified according to the five tastes, what organ they support, the degree of heat that they produce, the season that they should be consumed, and their effect on the movement of chi in the body.

FOOD AND THE FIVE ELEMENTS

	FIRE	EARTH	METAL	WATER	WOOD
Season	Summer	Indian summer	Autumn	Winter	Spring
Taste	Bitter	Sweet	Pungent/ spicy	Salty	Sour
Movement of Chi	Clears heat	Moistens and softens	Upward and outward	Downward and softening	Astringent
Spirit/Mind	Creativity	Intellect	Relationship with others	Willpower	Intuition, planning, and inspiration
Emotion	Cruelty, impatience versus love and joy	Anxiety versus openness and centeredness	Sadness versus courage	Fear versus gentleness	Anger versus kindness

The five tastes are bitter, sweet, salty, sour, and spicy. Each of these tastes has correspondences to aspects of the phenomenal world, to the extent that a balanced diet can help to create a balanced person. If your diet avoids the bitter taste, for example, you might ask yourself if you are avoiding issues around a balanced heart. Is there impatience or cruelty that requires recognition? An excessive sweet tooth may be associated with exhausted thinking. Within the principle of alchemy and Taoist realization, returning to the one means fusing equal aspects of energy from the five elements. Therefore all tastes must be explored. Discover and enjoy bitter, sour, and pungent just as much as sweet and salty, which are highly favored in our Western society. These tastes carry with them certain aspects of consciousness, so you can expand your mind by exploring the wonderful world of bitter and sour in vegetables, teas, meats, and condiments.

In the Tao of flavor, however, there is also a deep appreciation of the bland. Bland is the taste equivalent of peace. Quiet but full, the grains—such as barley, rye, and rice—provide that quiet center. Not all we eat needs to be extreme in flavor.

Each of the five flavors moves the body's chi in different ways—either expanding, contracting, lifting, descending, or centering it. Much of this movement occurs in the hours after digestion.

Cravings by definition imply a strong desire for the wrong food. In imbalanced states, the body will crave foods that may be temporarily soothing but harmful in the longer term. In spleen dampness or insufficiency, for example, the body can crave sugar for its soothing effects. The trouble is that the sugar injures the spleen even further, resulting in further weakness. Timing of meals can contribute to sugar cravings: if meals are not regular you can become overhungry and relatively hypoglycemic. Consequently, you will have cravings for sugars or other carbohydrates. The only way to get off the downward spiral is to forcibly abstain from sugars for a while, thereby allowing the spleen to recover.

Salt can create a similar spiral. Because salt helps agitated chi to descend, someone with excessive fear and insecurity may experience salt cravings. The salt will help settle the fears for a while, but excess salt damages the kidney, and a damaged kidney results in more fear.[12]

Craving for fat can be related to a student's desire "to feel secure, to slow down, and to have ample energy and warmth."[13] The trouble is that fats hurt the liver, creating dysfunction and clouding the spirit/ mind functions of planning and intuition. A disturbed liver also creates anger, which unsettles the person who then may seek more comfort from fatty foods.

Coffee stimulates the adrenals and damages kidney yin while exhausting kidney yang. While it gives a momentary feeling of excitement or energy, it soon creates the opposite effect. The reduced kidney yin means the liver heats up and the person can become irritable and angry. The loss of cooling power results in unopposed heart yang, so insomnia results.

Alcohol in small doses may be beneficial to health but for many it becomes a false goal. Calmness and connectedness need to be found by natural means. For many this is hard work. Some would rather sit and drink (or take drugs) than go through the discipline of attending classes and committing to practice. Alcohol in excess destroys kidney, heart, and lung yin while creating liver chi stagnation.[14] For many, gross imbalances in the body create cravings for relief. Therefore, to address these cravings the gross imbalances in lifestyle and diet need to be addressed first. An analysis of all taboo foods is beyond the confines of this text. Taboo foods include: sugar, honey, processed flour (biscuits, muffins), chocolate, and mainstream dairy products. Small amounts can be tolerated but significant portions will hurt the body.

Cooking, eating, and digestion can incorporate the other pillars of good health, if you allow meal time to become a ritual that celebrates your connections to loved ones, friends, and colleagues. Cook with love and the intention of healing. Food is medicinal and can thus be adapted to the needs of your family or friends. Invoke the magic of nature with alternating recipes dependent on the seasons. Don't forget to link the material food to the spiritual world: launch every meal with a blessing of the food.

Harmonizing with the Natural World

Eating the same food all the year round is possible in our modern societies, because food can be refrigerated and transported all around the world. However, this phenomenon denies the variety and balancing function that the earth and its seasons offer us. Each season is characterized by a certain external climate—warmth or coolness—that needs to be balanced in order to achieve homeostasis.

Foodstuffs are generated beneath the earth and water, just above the surface, and high in the trees; nearby creatures appear and disappear according to nature's patterns. Look to these natural variations to help you harmonize with nature. In summer, for example, eat more cooling raw foods and fruit off the trees. In winter eat those carbohydrate-rich roots from beneath the earth that warm us. In late spring eat the vegetables that rise and sit close to the earth. If you don't grow your own, then buy your produce from the market where local seasonal products are displayed. They look fresh and are usually cheaper. Of course, organic is best as pesticides, hormones, or synthetic chemicals imply an attempt to be discordant with nature. Food that has been stored and refrigerated has less chi than fresh produce.

In addition to eating with the seasons, it is important to vary your intake according to the rhythms of the daily cycle. According to Adelle Davis (1904–1974), an American nutritionist, we should "Eat breakfast like a king, lunch like a prince, and dinner like a pauper."[15] In our culture, most people do the exact opposite: breakfast is a bowl of processed cereal laced with sugar, coupled with toast and coffee. There is no preparation and all is carried out in haste. Lunch might be a sandwich, while dinner is generally the biggest and most prepared meal of the day.

The solution to this imbalance is not to reverse your habits overnight, but to get up a little bit earlier and have a cooked breakfast. At lunch time, attempt in some way to extract yourself from work. See the meal as a refuge of calm, and delight in its tastes. End with some time for digestion, which can include a walk or rest. (Many societies maintain at least two hours for lunch, so that there is time for a post-prandial nap.) Dinner becomes a light snack; expect to go to bed feeling a little light and hungry initially. After a while, you begin to enjoy that hungry feeling: meditation becomes easier and sleep becomes a creative endeavor—a source of creativity and new insights.

Traditional Chinese medicine (TCM) recognizes that one size does not fit all; individuals will need to vary their diets according to their constitutions and specific health issues. In Taoist thought, every human is made up of varying proportions of the five elements, each of which is intimately linked with the strength of an organ. Each person has strong and weak organs and can tailor his or her lifestyle to support the weak ones. Those with digestive/spleen weakness, for example, should avoid sugars and sweets, dairy products, raw foods, and sweet citrus. Those with liver stagnation or heat then should stay away from alcohol, coffee (regular or decaffeinated), heavy red meats, and spicy pungent foods. For those with excessive phlegm (respiratory conditions, bronchitis, sinusitis) avoid dairy, sweets, and fatty foods. If you have kidney weakness (bad back) avoid stimulants (caffeine), artificial sweeteners, and chilled foods. For deficiency states (chronic fatigue) eat regular small portions of meat, easily digestible (cooked) grains, cooked leafy greens, marrow broths, and soups. The list goes on, but the important common denominator is for each person to acknowledge her own individual constitution and develop a diet to promote healing.

In TCM the stomach is seen as a warm cook pot. Ingredients placed in it must be finely chopped, mixed, and prewarmed. Therefore the stomach needs the action of mastication to fragment foodstuffs into very small pieces and warm them up. It's important to chew your food to a watery consistency and to avoid icy cold drinks that negate the warming function of the stomach. Don't eat in a hurry, as this activates the sympathetic rather than the parasympathetic nervous system. Try not to read or watch television while eating; instead enjoy eating for all its pleasure.

Aids to digestion include aperitifs and appetizers. For those who abstain from alcohol, quality water with or without additives such as lemon juice can serve the same function. From a Western viewpoint, we want the parasympathetic nervous system and the digestive juices—including saliva—to be flowing well before the main meal. From a TCM perspective, the wetting, lubricating yin functions of the spleen must be encouraged.

Digestion plays a vital role in the body's health and should not be taken for granted.

Aid your digestive functions by enjoying some quiet time post meal, including a catnap. Others find a casual stroll promotes digestion and assists elimination. Treat yourself like a baby: encourage the food to go down by burping and rubbing your tummy. Often a small amount of sweet—a piece of fruit, for instance, which contains natural sugars—can quietly assist and soothe the spleen.

Healthy nutrition is just as much an art as science. It is important to test and investigate methods and foods in your own laboratory (your body) and observe how various things affect you. Be inspired by various texts and theories, but remember that the bottom line is how you feel and how your Tai Chi is progressing.

Much of the improvement in your health relies on the process of "undoing" rather than "doing": we make an effort to return to the original pattern—to partake in the commune of nature and all its variations. It is undoing because we are unraveling the negative effects of our industrialized and modern society. The aim is to live in this world yet return to our former glory. The mother earth was always in charge of all aspects of the menu; our mission now is to merely unfold and return. Now mentally float in emptiness and stillness, let go of worries, rest in nonaction, absorb primordial qi after midnight, practice healing exercises in a calm setting, support and nourish life without fail, take healthy food and efficacious herbs—if you do all this, then a hundred years of vigorous longevity are your proper due.[16]

REST AND SLEEP

Rest and sleep are a vital pillar of health and key components of take-home practice. According to Taoist thought, there are three states of mind: the state of being awake, the state of meditation, and the state of sleep. Ultimately, in realization of the Tao all three states merge into one consciousness. This process of merging is highlighted by Chuang Tsu's memorable quote:

> Once upon a time, I, Chuang Tsu, dreamed I was a butterfly flying happily here and there, enjoying life without knowing who I was. Suddenly I woke up and I was indeed Chuang Tsu. Did Chuang Tsu dream he was a butterfly, or did the butterfly dream he was Chuang Tsu?[17]

Sleep is more than recovery time—it is an opportunity for physical and emotional healing, spiritual development, creative thinking, and problem solving. Taoists prepare for sleep as they do for meditation, Tai Chi, or Chi Kung—by filling the body with chi and opening the meridians and tan tiens. The three basic practices that are recommended prior to sleep are stretching, the Six Healing Sounds, and meditation.

As mentioned above, going to bed slightly hungry or just on the light side of satiation is optimum. Certainly going to bed soon after a heavy meal is wrong: digestion and sleep are both yin functions that require whole-body energetic systems. They cannot be done simultaneously without some negative side effects, which can include nightmares, disturbed sleep, or even insomnia.

Stretching

Proper stretching—using a combination of muscle lengthening, mindful relaxation, and mindful breathing—can clear out stagnant accumulations of toxic chi and fill the body with healthy chi. This is largely a yin process that requires letting go and connecting to heaven and earth while providing a firm framework for the chi to enter. As energy levels are lower at the end of the day, stretches before sleep are usually performed on the ground.*

The Six Healing Sounds

Preparation for sleep should include the Six Healing Sounds practice, which identifies and transforms negative emotions. The body becomes emotionally positive and a connection is made between organs, their respective spirits, and the universe. This preparation helps to ensure that the sleep state will be far-reaching and creative, not bogged down by negative emotions.

Meditation

Sitting meditation prior to sleep should have limited expectations. The goal is to have a gentle meditation to encourage a pleasant and inviting feeling. Avoid the stronger energizing meditations of the Fusion and Kan and Li practices. At some point a natural sensation of sleepiness will overtake the body and mind.

Falling Asleep

At this stage, roll onto your side (preferably the right side) with the left hand on top of the upper thigh of a bent leg. The right hand is placed under the head or at second best under the pillow. Next give yourself some brief dream commands, such as "I want to come to a solution for the following problem in the morning," or "Please my spirit, venture out and solve this problem," or "Please give the answer to me as a thought in the morning or, alternatively, help me

---

*See Mantak Chia, *Energy Balance through the Tao*, (Rochester, Vt.: Destiny Books, 2005).

remember a relevant dream." The problem may be a chi blockage in your body that you are having difficulty clearing, excess yang and insufficient yin energies, or some other situation. Whatever the problem, ask your spirit and dream world for help.

Chen Tuan (871–989) was a Taoist sage who practiced on Hua Shan Mountain. According to legend he would sleep for months at a time with no signs of life. Vegetation would grow upon him. He understood sleeping habits this way:

> An ordinary person eats to satiation and then takes plenty of rest. He or she is mainly worried that the food should not be too rich, eating when he feels hungry and sleeping when he feels stirred. His snore is audible all over the place. Yet then at night, when he should be sound asleep, he wakes up unaccountably. This is because fame and gain, sounds and sights agitate his spirit and consciousness; sweet wine and fried mutton muddle his mind and will. This is the sleep of ordinary folk. But I practice the sleep of the perfected.[18]

Chen Tuan highlights one of the foundation principles of Taoism, which is that in order to find peace, the adept needs to let go of attachment to the external senses and to accomplishment. Instead, he needs to become eager and even fulfilled by the inner world of chi sensations and dreams. Chen Tuan's methodology involves a combination of lucid dreaming and alchemical practice. His book, *Xiandao Jing* (The Scripture That Manifests the Tao), describes meditations that can be carried out in the reclining position. These give us clues as to how to optimize our rest and sleep and to align ourselves with the Tao. These meditations can be done both day and night.[19]

Dream Practice

Practices are best performed in an isolated (close to nature) chamber that is clean and dry. Diet should be modified before practice so that solid food is reduced and a sense of lightness is obtained. This meditation is best done after bathing; the student can be nude or wear a light robe.

1. Begin by lying on your back. Focus your mind on the lower tan tien, then gather the spirit or essence of each organ and merge them in the lower tan tien.

    If you like, you can use a ritual incantation to summon the spirits residing in the organs. Do this by chanting their names in the order of the creation cycle: Houhou or Shen (heart), Beibei or Yi (spleen), Yanyan or Po (lungs), Fu Fu or Zhi (kidneys), and Jianjian or Hun (liver).[20]

2. Repeat the chanting and gathering until a bright light and warmth appear in the lower tan tien. Opening this place will automatically open the Microcosmic Orbit.

3. Coordinate your breathing with this meditation to assist the process: inhaling stimulates the kidneys and liver, while exhaling moves the heart and lungs to the centerpoint—the stomach and spleen.

Process the content of your dream during the day and, if necessary, take action in the material world.

⟳ Lucid Dreaming

To encourage lucid dreaming, bring the merged five spirits from the lower tan tien up to the heart and then to the Crystal Palace (also known as the Divine Palace or Hall of Light). The team of merged spirits can exit via the crown.

In general, the student's spirit should consciously explore the heavens and the earth, absorbing various essences and placing them in his cauldron. He should develop his practice to a stage where alchemical practices like Kan and Li and the Sealing of the Five Senses can be performed during sleep.

ALCHEMY

What began as the learning of a short Tai Chi sequence ends up encompassing all of our being! There are no shortcuts but to live in harmony with the Tao. Yet for every time you feel overwhelmed by the work that needs to be done in this life, you will have the joy of progress.

Progress is an individual experience, so to compare yourself to others is irrelevant. Chang San-Feng encourages us each to make our unique contribution when he says, "No matter whether brilliant or foolish, virtuous or otherwise, all can use their innate knowledge and abilities to approach the Tao."[21] The internal martial arts are fun and are there to be enjoyed. There will always be others more skilled at external tricks such as Fa Jin and Iron Shirt; remember that these tricks are not an endpoint. Develop your own skill to the level that is right for you. Don't be distracted; stay on track!

Tai Chi can be regarded as an internal alchemy whose movements and forces provide a material platform for spiritual forces. To understand this, imagine a spirit being who wishes to escape the boredom of heavenly existence. Then imagine an earthbound soul who yearns to escape the earthly plane and its material sufferings. The only solution is to master and marry both levels of existence and return to the unity that is the Tao.

The reader will soon realize that ultimate competence in Tai Chi requires us to infuse the body and movement with the immaterial phenomena of chi, jin, and spirit. This can only be accomplished by mastering all aspects of our physical, emotional, and spiritual being.

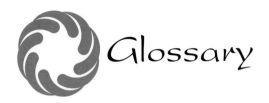# Glossary

An: one of the eight gates—Push or water power

Ba Fa Jin: eight gates of discharge power

Ba Gua/Pakua: eight-sided symbol representing the eight forces of nature

Ba Hui: crown of the head point

Bei Bei: thinking spirit of the spleen, also see Yi

chan su jin: silk reeling

chi: the vibration of the life force felt by the senses

Chi Kung: to work the chi

Ching Chi: fluid essence most commonly associated with sexual essence

Chong Mai: Central Thrusting Channel

Chou: one of the eight gates—Elbow Strike

Dai Mai: Belt Channel

Du Mai: Governing Channel

dong jin: understanding power

empty force: Spontaneous movement and contraction of muscle groups that occurs in the setting of relaxation and exhalation

fa song: relaxing and filling the body with chi

Fa Jin: internal discharge power

Fu Fu: see Zhi

Hou-Hou: see Shen

Hun: the liver's ethereal soul

Jian Jian: see Hun

Ji: one of the eight gates—Press or bounce power

jin: internal power

Jing Well Points: distal points of the acupuncture meridians on the fingers and toes

kan, li, zheng, tui, kun, ken, sun, chien: water, fire, thunder, lake, earth, mountain, wind, and heaven

kang: resisting

Kou: one of the eight gates—the Shoulder Strike

ku: food chi

kua: the ligaments of the pelvis

Li power: Using external muscular strength rather than chi or jin power

Lieh: one of the eight gates—splitting power

Lu: one of the eight gates—Rollback

Ming Men: Door of Life point, between the second and third lumbar vertebrae

mudra: positioning of the body to hasten flow of chi or invoke spiritual power

Nei Kung: internal strength work

Ni Chan: yang aspect of Fa Jin

Peng: one of the eight gates—Ward Off or spring power

Po: the lung's corporeal soul

Pu: the state of simplicity, the "uncarved block" indicative of the Wu Wei

Radial: forearm bone on the thumb side

Ren Mai: Conception Channel

ruan: limp rather than fa song

Shu Chan: yin aspect of Fa Jin

Shen: spirit that resides in the heart

sung: see fa song

synovial fluid: the lubricating fluid in joints

tan tien: energy center

ting jin: listening power

Tsai: one of the eight gates—lever power

Tui Shou: Push Hands

ulna: forearm bone

vestibular system: balance center of the inner ear

Yao: the waist, including the lower tan tien

Yi: integrated mind power, also the thinking spirit of the spleen

Wu Wei: nothingness

Xu Jin: collection of power

Yan Yan: see Po

ying: excessively hard, using Li power

zhan, lian, nian, sui: connecting, sticking, adhering, and following

Zhi: willpower from the kidneys

Cast of Taoist/Tai Chi Characters
(See chapter 1 for more details)

Chang San-Feng (1279–1368 CE): legendary immortal who created Tai Chi

Chen Man-Ching (1902–1975): student of Yang Chen-Fu

Chen Tuan (871–989): Taoist sage who perfected sleeping

Chen Tin-Hung (1930–2005): Southern Wu style master (renamed Wu Tang style)

Chen Wan-Ting (1628–1736): founder of Chen style Tai Chi

Chuang Tsu (4th century BCE): greatest Chinese philosopher of all times

Dong Hai-Chuan (1797–1882): founder of Ba Gua Zhang

Ken Yue-Kwong (Rocky) (1934–   ): Southern Wu style master

Lee, Bruce (1940–1973): movie star

Li Bing-Ci (1929–   ): Northern Wu style master

Li I-Yu (1832–1892): taught by Wu Yu-Hsiang

Lao Tsu (sixth century BCE): founder of Taoism and author of Tao Te Ching

Ma Yueh-Liang (1901–1999): husband of Wu Ying-Hua

Sun Lu-Tang (1861–1932): founder of the Sun style Tai Chi

Tan Meng-Hsien: little is known except included in Yang family manuscripts

Wang Mao-Zhai (1862–1940): grandfather of the Northern Wu style

Wang Pei-Sheng (1919–2004): Northern Wu style master

Wang Tsung-Yueh (1812–1880): the first historical Tai Chi character after Chang San-Feng

Wu Gong-Tsao (1902–1983): son of Wu Jian-Chuan

Wu Jian-Chuan (1870–1942): son of Wu Chuan-Yu

Wu Chuan-Yu (1834–1902): founder of Wu style

Wu Tu-Nan (1884–1987): Wu master of the Northern school

Wu Ying-Hua (1907–1996): daughter of Wu Jian-Chuan

Wu Yu-Hsiang (1812–1880): founder of Hao style, taught by Yang Lu-Chan

Yang Chen-Fu (1883–1936): son of Yang Jian

Yang Jian (1839–1917): son of Yang-Lu Chan

Yang Lu-Chan (1799–1872): founder of the Yang style

Yang Pan-Hou (1837–1892): son of Yang Lu-Chan

Yee, Eddie: Master Chia's Wu style teacher

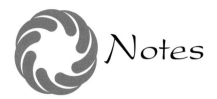

Notes

Chapter 1. History of the Wu Style

1. Peter Lim, *Tian Tek: Taijiquan's Resource Page*, January 15, 1998, www
   .itcca.it/peterlim/historg6.htm; viewed June 2010.
2. Wen Zee, *Wu Style Tai Chi Chuan: Ancient Chinese Way to Health* (Berkeley, Calif.: North Atlantic Books, 2002), 19.
3. Lim, *Tian Tek: Taijiquan's Resource Page*.
4. Christopher Majka, www.chebucto.ns.ca/Philosophy/Taichi/wu.html;
   viewed July 2010.
5. Yang Jun, *International Yang Family Tai Chi Chuan Association*, www
   .yangfamilytaichi.com/yang/history/#yang-shao-hou; viewed June 2010.
6. Tina Zhang and Frank Allen, *Classical Northern Wu Style Tai Ji Quan: The
   Fighting Art of the Manchurian Palace Guard* (Berkeley, Calif.: Blue Snake
   Books, 2006), 15.
7. Zhang Wen-Guang, Li Bin-Ci, et al., *Competition Routines for Four
   Styles Taijiquan* (Beijing: People's Sports Publishing House of China,
   1991), 3.
8. Zhang and Allen, *Classical Northern Wu Style Tai Ji Quan*, 39.
9. Chu Man-Sit Association, www.taihui.com/history.html; viewed December 2010.
10. Cheng Tin-Hung and D. J. Docherty, *Wu Tan Tai Chi Chuan* (Hong
    Kong: D. J. Docherty, 1983), 31.

Chapter 2. Why Practice Wu Style Tai Chi Chi Kung?

1. Wu Grand Master Wu Tu-Nan in Wang Pei-Sheng and Zeng Wei-Qi,
   *Wu Style Taijiquan: A Detailed Course for Health and Self Defence and Teach-
   ings of Three Famous Masters in Beijing* (Hong Kong: Hai Feng Publishing
   Co., 1983), 223.
2. Wang Chen-Chen and Lean-Paul Collet, "The Effect of Tai Chi on

Health Outcomes in Patients with Chronic Conditions: A Systematic Review," *Archives of Internal Medicine* 164 (March 2004): 500.

3. Ibid.

4. Ruth Taylor-Piliae, "Tai Chi as an Adjunct to Cardiac Rehabilitation Exercise Training: A Review Article," *Journal of Cardiopulmonary Rehabilitation* 23 (2003): 91.

5. A. Han, M. Judd, et al., "Tai Chi for Treating Rheumatoid Arthritis," *Cochrane Database of Systematic Reviews* 3 (2004), CD004849. DOI: 10.1002/14651858.CD004849.

6. Alice Kuramoto, "Therapeutic Benefits of Tai Chi: A Systematic Review," *Wisconsin Medical Journal* 105, no. 7 (2006): 46.

7. Paul Lam, "Variation in Speed," *Tai Chi Health and Lifestyle Newsletter* May 2003, in Michael P. Garofalo, "Cloud Hands Website," www .egreenway.com/taichichuan/chenquote.htm#Quotes; viewed January 25, 2010. Dr. Paul Lam is a medical practitioner in Sydney, Australia. He is an accomplished Tai Chi practitioner, becoming winner of Beijing 42 and second place in the Chen style forms at the Third International Tai Chi Competition in Beijing.

8. Chang San-Feng, "Tai Chi Chuan Ching," in *The Essence of Tai Chi Chuan: The Literary Tradition*, ed. Benjamin Lo and Martin Inn (Berkeley, Calif.: North Atlantic Books, 1979), 25.

9. Wu Gong-Tsao, "Lecture of Taijiquan," in *Tai Chi Secrets of the Wu Style*, trans. and comm. Yang Jwing-Ming (Boston: YMAA Publications, 2002), 1.

10. Sun Lu-Tang, *Study of Taiji Boxing* (1921), quoted in Joseph Crandall, *Taijiquan Xue* (2000), 6. Quoted on *Cloud Hands Website*, www .egreenway.com/taichichuan/sunquotes1.htm#Crandall1; viewed January 25, 2010.

Chapter 3. Wu Style Principles

1. Wu Gong-Tsao, "Lecture of Taijiquan," in *Tai Chi Secrets of the Wu Style*, trans. and comm. Yang Jwing-Ming (Boston: YMAA Publications, 2002), 61.

2. Wang Pei-Sheng and Zeng Wei-Qi, *Wu Style Taijiquan: A Detailed Course for Health and Self Defence and Teachings of Three Famous Masters in Beijing* (Hong Kong: Hai Feng Publishing Co., 1983), 215.

3. Yang Chen-Fu, "The Ten Important Points for Tai Chi Chuan," in *T'ai-*

chi Touchstones: Yang Family Secret Transmissions, trans. and ed. Douglas Wile (Brooklyn, New York: Sweet Ch'i Press, 1983), 12.

4. Wang Pei-Sheng and Zeng Wei-Qi, *Wu Style Taijiquan*, 215.

5. Wen Zee, *Wu Style Tai Chi Chuan: Ancient Chinese Way to Health* (Berkeley, Calif.: North Atlantic Books, 2002), 118.

6. Yang Chen-Fu, "The Ten Important Points for Tai Chi Chuan," in *T'ai-chi Touchstones*, trans. and ed. Wile, 12.

7. Wu Yu-Hsiang, "Expositions of Insights into the Practice of the Thirteen Postures," in *The Essence of Tai Chi Chuan: The Literary Tradition*, ed. Benjamin Lo and Martin Inn (Berkeley, Calif.: North Atlantic Books, 1979), 49.

8. Marnix Wells, trans., and Chang Naizhou, *Scholar Boxer: Chang Naizhou's Theory of Internal Martial Arts and the Evolution of Taijiquan* (Berkeley, Calif.: North Atlantic Books, 2005), 64.

9. Wen Zee, *Wu Style Tai Chi Chuan*, 119.

10. Ma Hai-Long, *About Jin-Power*, trans. Lukas Kasenda, www.wu-taichi.com/About; viewed November 2010.

11. Wu Gong-Tsao, "Lecture of Taijiquan," in *Tai Chi Secrets*, trans. and comm. Yang Jwing-Ming, 23.

12. Davidine Sim and David Gaffney, *Chen Style Taijiquan: The Source of Taiji Boxing* (Berkeley, Calif.: North Atlantic Books, 2002), 163.

13. Yang Pan-Hou, "Yang Family Forty Chapters," in *Lost T'ai-Ch'i Classics from the Late Ch'ing Dynasty*, trans. and ed. Douglas Wile (Albany: State University of New York Press, 1996), 66.

14. Ibid., 67.

15. Wu Yu-Hsiang, "Expositions of Insights," in *The Essence of Tai Chi Chuan*, ed. Lo and Inn, 53.

16. Ibid., 47.

17. See "The Oral Transmission of Zhang [Chang] San-Feng" in *Lost T'ai-Ch'i Classics*, trans. and ed. Wile, 87.

18. Wu Gong-Tsao, "Lecture of Taijiquan," in *Tai Chi Secrets*, trans. and comm. Yang Jwing-Ming, 27.

19. Yang Pan-Hou, "Yang Family Forty Chapters," in *Lost Tai-Ch'i Classics*, trans. and ed. Wile, 78.

20. Wu Gong-Tsao, "Lecture of Taijiquan," in *Tai Chi Secrets*, trans. and comm. Yang Jwing-Ming, 7.

21. Wu Yu-Hsiang, "Exposition of Insights into the Thirteen Postures,"

in *The Taijiquan Classics*, trans. and ed. Barbara Davis (Berkeley, Calif.: North Atlantic Books, 2004), 79.

22. Chang San-Feng, "Tai Chi Chuan Ching," in *The Essence of Tai Chi Chuan: The Literary Tradition*, ed. Benjamin Lo and Martin Inn (Berkeley, Calif.: North Atlantic Books, 1979), 19.

23. Erle Montaigue, *The Physical Side of the Internal Fighting Systems*, vol. 19, DVD MTG334. Available at www.taijiworld.com/Videos.

24. Wu Yu-Hsiang, "Expositions of Insights," in *The Taijiquan Classics*, trans. and ed. Davis, 79.

25. Wang Pei-Sheng and Zeng Wei-Qi, *Wu Style Taijiquan*, 8.

Chapter 4. Wu Style Warm-Ups

1. Robert and Marilyn Kriegel, *The C Zone: Peak Performance Under Pressure* (Garden City, N.Y.: Anchor Press/Doubleday, 1984), 2.

2. Chang San-Feng, "Taijiquan Jing," in *The Taijiquan Classics*, trans. and ed. Barbara Davis (Berkeley, Calif.: North Atlantic Books, 2004), 75.

3. Wu Gong-Tsao, "Lecture of Taijiquan," in *Tai Chi Secrets of the Wu Style*, trans. and comm. Yang Jwing-Ming (Boston: YMAA Publications, 2002), 3.

4. Ibid. 27.

5. Yang Pan-Hou, "Yang Family Forty Chapters" in *Lost T'ai-Ch'i Classics from the Late Ch'ing Dynasty*, trans. and ed. Douglas Wile (Albany: State University of New York Press, 1996), 77.

6. Ma Yueh-Liang and Wen Zee, *Wu Style Taichichuan Push Hands (Tuishou)* (Hong Kong: Shanghai Book Co., 1990), 22.

7. Lee Tin-Chan, *The Wu Style of Tai Chi Chuan* (Burbank, Calif.: Unique Publications, 1982), 10.

8. Wu Yu-Hsiang, "Expositions of Insights into the Practice of the Thirteen Postures," in *The Essence of Tai Chi Chuan: The Literary Tradition*, ed. Benjamin Lo and Martin Inn (Berkeley, Calif.: North Atlantic Books, 1979), 57.

9. Lao Tsu, *Tao Te Ching*, in *Tao Te Ching*, trans. Gia Feng and Jane English (New York: Vintage Books, Random House, 1972), chapter 16.

10. Chen Xin's works are described in *Scholar Boxer: Chang Naizhou's Theory of Internal Martial Arts and the Evolution of Taijiquan*, trans. Marnix Wells (Berkeley, Calif.: North Atlantic Books, 2005), 27.

11. Wang Pei-Sheng and Zeng Wei-Qi, *Wu Style Taijiquan: A Detailed Course*

for Health and Self Defence and Teachings of Three Famous Masters in Beijing (Hong Kong: Hai Feng Publishing Co., 1983), 6.

12. Davidine Siaw-Voon Sim and David Gaffney, *Chen Style Taijiquan: The Source of Taiji Boxing* (Berkeley, Calif.: North Atlantic Books, 2002), 46.

13. Li Yi-Yu, "Song of the Essence and Application of Tai Chi Chuan," in *Lost T'ai-Ch'i Classics from the Late Ching Dynasty*, trans. and ed. Douglas Wile (Albany: State University of New York Press, 1996), 50.

14. Wu Gong-Tsao, "Lecture of Taijiquan," in *Tai Chi Secrets*, trans. and comm. Yang Jwing-Ming, 15.

15. Tan Meng-Hsien, "Songs of the Eight Ways," in *T'ai-chi Touchstones: Yang Family Secret Transmissions*, trans. and ed. Douglas Wile (Brooklyn, New York: Sweet Ch'i Press, 1983), 28–35.

16. Ibid., 32.

17. Wu Gong-Tsao, "Lecture of Taijiquan," in *Tai Chi Secrets*, trans. and comm. Yang Jwing-Ming, 18.

18. Ibid., 20.

Chapter 7. Martial Applications of the Wu Style Form

1. Wang Pei-Sheng and Zeng Wei-Qi, *Wu Style Taijiquan: A Detailed Course for Health and Self Defence and Teachings of Three Famous Masters in Beijing* (Hong Kong: Hai Feng Publishing Co., 1983), 75–76.

Chapter 8. The Wu Style Tai Chi Boxing System

1. Wu Yu-Hsiang, "Expositions of Insights into the Practice of the Thirteen Postures," in *The Essence of Tai Chi Chuan: The Literary Tradition*, ed. Benjamin Lo and Martin Inn (Berkeley, Calif.: North Atlantic Books, 1979), 53.

2. Wu Gong-Tsao, "Lecture of Taijiquan," in *Tai Chi Secrets of the Wu Style*, trans. and comm. Yang Jwing-Ming (Boston: YMAA Publications, 2002), 21.

3. Ibid., 4.

4. Chang [Zhang] San-Feng, "Yang's Forty Chapters," in *Lost T'ai-Ch'i Classics from the Late Ching Dynasty*, trans. and ed. Douglas Wile (Albany: State University of New York Press, 1996), 87.

Chapter 9. Home Practice

1. Wu Gong-Tsao, "Lecture of Taijiquan," in *Tai Chi Secrets of the Wu*

Style, trans. and comm. Yang Jwing-Ming (Boston: YMAA Publications, 2002), 1.

2. Lao-Tse, *Tao Te Ching*, trans. James Legge (Thousand Oaks, Calif.: BN Publishing, 2007), chapter 44.

3. Chang San-Feng, "Taijiquan Jing," in *The Taijiquan Classics*, trans. and ed. Barbara Davis (Berkeley, Calif.: North Atlantic Books, 2004), 75.

4. Wu Yu-Hsiang, "Expositions of Insights into the Practice of the Thirteen Postures," in *The Essence of Tai Chi Chuan: The Literary Tradition*, ed. Benjamin Lo and Martin Inn (Berkeley, Calif.: North Atlantic Books, 1979), 57.

5. Wu Yu-Hsiang, "Expositions of Insights into the Practice of the Thirteen Postures," in *The Taijiquan Classics*, trans. and ed. Barbara Davis (Berkeley, Calif.: North Atlantic Books, 2004), 79.

6. *The Plain Dao of the Xiandao Jing: An Early Medieval Method of Reclining Meditation*, trans. Stephen Eskilden, Sixth International Conference on Daoist Studies, Conference Paper (LA 2010).

7. Wu Gong-Tsao, "Lecture of Taijiquan," in *Tai Chi Secrets*, trans. and comm. Yang Jwing-Ming, 1.

8. Leon Hammer, *Dragon Rises, Red Bird Flies: Psychology and Chinese Medicine* (Wellingborough, U.K.: Crucible, 1990), 104–12.

9. Ibid., 152.

10. Ibid., 148.

11. Don Colbert, *The Seven Pillars of Good Health* (Lake Mary, Fla.: Siloam, 2007).

12. Paul Pitchford, *Healing with Whole Foods: Oriental Traditions and Modern Nutrition* (Berkeley, Calif.: North Atlantic Books, 1993), 158.

13. Ibid., 119.

14. Ibid., 390.

15. http://adelledavis.org/quotations.

16. Yangxing Yanming Lu, quoted in Livia Kohn, *Daoist Dietetics: Food for Immortality* (Dunedin, Fla.: Three Pines Press, 2010), 71.

17. Chuang Tsu, *Inner Chapters*, trans. Gia-Fu Feng and Jane English (New York: Vintage Books, 1974), 48.

18. Chen Tuan, "Comprehensive Mirror Through the Ages of Perfected Immortals and Those Who Embody the Tao," in *The Taoist Experience: An Anthology*, ed. Livia Kohn (Albany, N.Y.: SUNY, 1983), 273; and Man-

tak Chia, *Sealing of the Five Senses: Opening of the Crystal Room* (Chiang Mai, Thailand: Universal Tao Publications, 2005).

19. *The Plain Dao of the Xiandao Jing*, trans. Eskilden.

20. Ibid.

21. Chang [Zhang] San-Feng, "Yang's Forty Chapters," in *Lost T'ai-Ch'i Classics from the Late Ching Dynasty*, trans. and ed. Douglas Wile (Albany: State University of New York Press, 1996), 88.

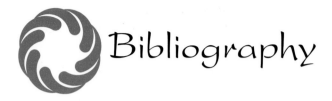# Bibliography

Cheng Tin-Hung, and D. J. Docherty. *Wu Tan Tai Chi Chuan*. Hong Kong: D. J. Docherty, 1983.

Chan Wing-Tsit, trans. *A Sourcebook in Chinese Philosophy*. Princeton, NJ: Princeton University Press, 1963.

Chuang Tsu. *Inner Chapters: A Companion Volume to Tao Te Ching*. Translated by Gia-Fu Feng and Jane English. New York: Vintage Books, 2000.

Colbert, Don. *The Seven Pillars of Good Health*. Lake Mary, Fla.: Siloam, 2007.

Davis, Barbara, trans and ed. *The Taijiquan Classics*. Berkeley, Calif.: North Atlantic Books, 2004.

Emery, Adrian. *The Art of Nourishment*. Hallidays Point, NSW, Australia: Blackhead Ink, 1993.

Flaws, Bob, and Honora Wolfe. *Prince Wen Hui's Cook: Chinese Dietary Therapy*. Brookline, Mass.: Paradigm, 1983.

Flaws, Bob. *Arisal of the Clear: A Simple Guide to Healthy Eating According to Traditional Chinese Medicine*. Boulder, Colo.: Blue Poppy, 1991.

Frantzis, Bruce Kumar. *The Power of Internal Martial Arts and Chi: Combat and Energy Secrets of Bagua, Tai Chi and Hsing Yi*. California: Energy Arts, 2007.

Han, A., M. Judd, et al. "Tai Chi for Treating Rheumatoid Arthritis." *Cochrane Database of Systematic Reviews* 3 (2004), CD004849. DOI: 10.1002/14651858.CD004849.

Hammer, Leon. *Dragon Rises, Red Bird Flies: Psychology and Chinese Medicine*. Wellingborough, U.K.: Crucible, 1990.

Kohn, Livia. *Daoist Dietetics: Food for Immortality*. Dunedin, Fla.: Three Pines Press, 2010.

———, ed. *The Taoist Experience: An Anthology*. Albany, N.Y.: SUNY, 1983.

Kriegel, Robert, and Marilyn Kriegel. *The C Zone: Peak Performance Under Pressure*. Garden City, N.Y.: Anchor Press/Doubleday, 1984.

Kuo Lien-Ying. *The Tai Chi Boxing Chronicle*. Translated by Gordon Guttmann. Berkeley, Calif.: North Atlantic Books, 1994.

Kuramoto, Alice. "Therapeutic Benefits of Tai Chi: A Systematic Review." *Wisconsin Medical Journal* 105, no. 7 (2006): 42–46.

Lee Tin-Chan. *The Wu Style of Tai Chi Chuan*. Burbank, Calif.: Unique Publications, 1982.

Lao-Tse. *Tao Te Ching*. Translated by James Legge. Thousand Oaks, Calif.: BN Publishing, 2007.

———. *Tao Te Ching*. Translated by Gia-Fu Feng and Jane English. New York: Vintage Books, 1972.

Lo, Benjamin, and Martin Inn, eds. *The Essence of Tai Chi Chuan: The Literary Tradition*. Berkeley, Calif.: North Atlantic Books, 1979.

Lu, Henry. *Chinese System of Food Cures: Prevention and Remedies*. New York: Sterling, 1986.

Ma Yueh-Liang and Zee Wen. *Wu Style Taichichuan Push Hands (Tuishou)*. Hong Kong: Shanghai Book Co., 1990.

Pitchford, Paul. *Healing with Whole Foods: Oriental Traditions and Modern Nutrition*. Berkeley, Calif.: North Atlantic Books, 1993.

Sim, Davidine Siaw Voon, and David Gaffney. *Chen Style Taijiquan: The Source of Taiji Boxing*. Berkeley, Calif.: North Atlantic Books, 2002.

Taylor-Piliae, Ruth E. "Tai Chi as an Adjunct to Cardiac Rehabilitation Exercise Training: A Review Article." *Journal of Cardiopulmonary Rehabilitation* 23 (2003): 90–96.

Wang Chen-Chen and Jean Paul Collet. "The Effect of Tai Chi on Health Outcomes in Patients with Chronic Conditions: A Systematic Review." *Archives of Internal Medicine* 164 (March 2004): 493–501.

Wang Pei-Sheng and Zeng Wei-Qi. *Wu Style Taijiquan: A Detailed Course for Health and Self Defence and Teachings of Three Famous Masters in Beijing*. Hong Kong: Hai Feng Publishing Co., 1983.

Wells, Marnix, trans., and Chang Naizhou. *Scholar Boxer: Chang Naizhou's Theory of Internal Martial Arts and the Evolution of Taijiquan*. Berkeley, Calif.: North Atlantic Books, 2005.

Wile, Douglas, trans. and ed., *T'ai-chi Touchstones: Yang Family Secret Transmissions*. Brooklyn, New York: Sweet Ch'i Press, 1983.

———, trans. and ed. *Lost T'ai-Ch'i Classics from the Late Ch'ing Dynasty*. Albany: State University of New York Press, 1996.

————. *T'ai-Chi's Ancestors: The Making of an Internal Martial Art.* Brooklyn, New York: Sweet Ch'i Press, 1999.

Yang Jwing-Ming, trans. and comm. *Tai Chi Secrets of the Wu Style.* Boston: YMAA Publications, 2002.

————. *Tai Chi Secrets of the Yang Styles.* Boston: YMAA Publications, 2001.

————. *Tai Chi Secrets of the Wu and Li Styles.* Boston: YMAA Publications, 2001.

Zee, Wen. *Wu Style Tai Chi Chuan: Ancient Chinese Way to Health.* Berkeley, Calif.: North Atlantic Books, 2002.

Zhang, Tina Chunna, and Frank Allen. *Classical Northern Wu Style Tai Ji Quan: The Fighting Art of the Manchurian Palace Guard.* Berkeley, Calif.: Blue Snake Books, 2006.

Zhang Wen-Guang, Li Bin-Ci, et al. *Competition Routines for Four Styles Taijiquan.* Beijing: People's Sports Publishing House of China, 1991.

Websites

www.northernwutaijiquan.com
www.metal-tiger.com/Wu_Tang_PCA/NorthernWu.html
www.chebucto.ns.ca/Philosophy/Taichi/wu.html
www.itcca.it/peterlim/historg6.htm
www.wu-taichi.de/cms/wu-taichi.com/index

About the Authors

MANTAK CHIA

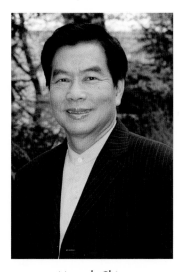

Mantak Chia

Mantak Chia has been studying the Taoist approach to life since childhood. His mastery of this ancient knowledge, enhanced by his study of other disciplines, has resulted in the development of the Universal Healing Tao system, which is now being taught throughout the world.

Mantak Chia was born in Thailand to Chinese parents in 1944. When he was six years old, he learned from Buddhist monks how to sit and "still the mind." While in grammar school he learned traditional Thai boxing, and he soon went on to acquire considerable skill in aikido, yoga, and Tai Chi. His studies of the Taoist way of life began in earnest when he was a student in Hong Kong, ultimately leading to his mastery of a wide variety of esoteric disciplines, with the guidance of several masters, including Master I Yun, Master Meugi, Master Cheng Yao Lun, and Master Pan Yu. To better understand the mechanisms behind healing energy, he also studied Western anatomy and medical sciences.

Master Chia has taught his system of healing and energizing

practices to tens of thousands of students and trained more than two thousand instructors and practitioners throughout the world. He has established centers for Taoist study and training in many countries around the globe. In June of 1990, he was honored by the International Congress of Chinese Medicine and Qi Gong (Chi Kung), which named him the Qi Gong Master of the Year.

ANDREW JAN

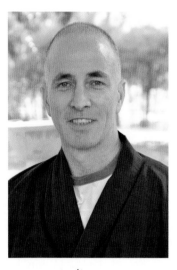

Andrew Jan

Dr. Andrew Jan is a senior instructor for the Universal Healing Tao system. He first became an instructor in 1992 and has been a senior instructor since 2001. He began studying martial arts as a young child and has been studying the internal arts of Wu Shu for twenty-five years. His teachers include: Chen Lu, John Yuen (Blackburn Tai Chi Academy), Liu De-Ming (Associate Professor Martial Arts, Fujien University), Liu Hong-Chi (Beijing), Huo Dong-Li (Senior Judge, Beijing Wu Shu Federation), Zhu Tian-Cai (one of the contemporary "tigers" of Chen Jia Guo), and of course Master Mantak Chia.

Dr. Andrew Jan has won multiple medals in Push Hands competitions and a Full-Contact All Styles Lightweight Division in 1984 in Victoria. In 2000, he became the National Tai Chi and Wu Shu Champion in the over-40 section, and also won first place in Wu Style, Yang Style, and Weapon divisions.

Dr. Andrew Jan is currently practicing as an Emergency Medicine Physician and Medical Acupuncturist. He also runs a private medical practice where he integrates Chinese and Western medicine. He has a bachelor's degree in the arts as well as a master's degree in philosophy. Dr. Andrew Jan was born in Australia to a Chinese father and an English mother. He has always found himself exploring and synthesizing Eastern and Western traditions, an ability he applies to healing as well as martial arts. He has to date coauthored four books with Mantak Chia on Tai Chi and advanced Taoist meditation. He is married to his loving wife and fellow practitioner, Fiona, with one daughter, Nikita.

The Universal Healing Tao System and Training Center

THE UNIVERSAL HEALING TAO SYSTEM

The ultimate goal of Taoist practice is to transcend physical boundaries through the development of the soul and the spirit within the human. That is also the guiding principle behind the Universal Tao, a practical system of self-development that enables individuals to complete the harmonious evolution of their physical, mental, and spiritual bodies. Through a series of ancient Chinese meditative and internal energy exercises, the practitioner learns to increase physical energy, release tension, improve health, practice self-defense, and gain the ability to heal him- or herself and others. In the process of creating a solid foundation of health and well-being in the physical body, the practitioner also creates the basis for developing his or her spiritual potential by learning to tap into the natural energies of the sun, moon, earth, stars, and other environmental forces.

The Universal Tao practices are derived from ancient techniques rooted in the processes of nature. They have been gathered and integrated into a coherent, accessible system for well-being that works directly with the life force, or chi, that flows through the meridian system of the body.

286

Master Chia has spent years developing and perfecting techniques for teaching these traditional practices to students around the world through ongoing classes, workshops, private instruction, and healing sessions, as well as books and video and audio products. Further information can be obtained at www.universal-tao.com.

THE UNIVERSAL TAO TRAINING CENTER

The Tao Garden Resort and Training Center in northern Thailand is the home of Master Chia and serves as the worldwide headquarters for Universal Tao activities. This integrated wellness, holistic health, and training center is situated on eighty acres surrounded by the beautiful Himalayan foothills near the historic walled city of Chiang Mai. The serene setting includes flower and herb gardens ideal for meditation, open-air pavilions for practicing Chi Kung, and a health and fitness spa.

The center offers classes year round, as well as summer and winter retreats. It can accommodate two hundred students, and group leasing can be arranged. For information worldwide on courses, books, products, and other resources, see below.

RESOURCES

Universal Healing Tao Center
274 Moo 7, Luang Nua, Doi Saket, Chiang Mai, 50220 Thailand
Tel: (66)(53) 495-596 Fax: (66)(53) 495-852
E-mail: universaltao@universal-tao.com
Website: www.universal-tao.com

For information on retreats and the health spa, contact:
Tao Garden Health Spa & Resort
E-mail: info@tao-garden.com, taogarden@hotmail.com
Website: www.tao-garden.com

Good Chi • Good Heart • Good Intention

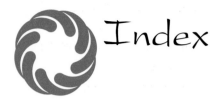 # Index

Page numbers in *italics* represent illustrations.